# CRITICAL MASS

## The Positions-Of-Flexion Approach to Explosive Muscle Growth

by Steve Holman
Photography by Michael Neveux

*IRONMAN's CRITICAL MASS* was written to help you reach your physical potential with sensible bodybuilding training strategies. Weight training is a demanding activity, however, so it is highly recommended that you consult your physician and have a physical examination prior to beginning a weight-training program. Proceed with the suggested exercises and routines at your own risk.

IRONMAN *would like to extend special thanks to the bodybuilders whose images appear in this book: Paul DeMayo, Tom Varga, Roger Stewart, Frank Hillebrand, Franco Santoriello, Michael Ashley, Gary Strydom, Brian Buchanan, Chris Duffy, Mark Rollins, Robby Robinson, Lionel Rangel, Lee Labrada, Ray McNeil, Thierry Pastel and Vince Taylor.*

Cover design by Leon Bach

**ISBN 0-9627834-2-0**
**Library of Congress Catalog Card Number: 94-96142**

Copyright © 1994 by *IRONMAN* Magazine
All rights reserved.

The material in this document may not be reproduced in whole or in part in any manner or form without prior written consent from the publisher.

**IRONMAN Publishing**
1701 Ives Ave., Oxnard, CA 93033

# CONTENTS

**FOREWORD**..................................................................11

**INTRODUCTION**............................................................15

**1 CRITICAL CALVES**
    *A No-Bull Approach for Mass Below the Knees*..................19

**2 CRITICAL QUADS AND HAMS**
    *Build Tree-Trunk-Size Thighs*...........................................29

**3 CRITICAL CHEST**
    *The Quest for Pec Perfection*..........................................41

**4 CRITICAL BACK**
    *Building a Back That's Wide, Thick and Majestic*...............51

**5 CRITICAL DELTS**
    *A Boulder Approach*......................................................63

**6 CRITICAL ARMS**
    *Shoulder-to-Wrist Growth Blitz*........................................71

**7 CRITICAL ABDOMINALS**
    *A New Approach to Rippling Ruggedness*.......................85

**8 POF EVERY-OTHER-DAY SPLIT**....................................93

**9 POF HARDGAINER ROUTINE**.......................................99

**10 POF POWER PROGRAM**............................................105

**11 POF TARGET OVERLOAD**..........................................111

**12 POF PRE-EXHAUSTION**.............................................117

**AFTERWORD**................................................................123

# FOREWORD

New techniques that spur higher levels of sports performance often emerge after logical study. Bob Fosbury, a high jumper in the '60s, was the creator of just such a technique. He studied the universally practiced method of hurdling the high bar, analyzed the physics involved and developed a better way—launching the body backward, going over the bar headfirst. It was called the Fosbury Flop, and with it he set an amazing world-record jump at the '68 Olympics in Mexico, surprising the athletic community and coming away with a gold medal. Today all high jumpers use Fosbury's method.

A more recent example occurred in swimming. For years coaches believed that swimmers got the maximum propulsion through the water while keeping their fingers together. After careful observation, however, the experts discovered that when the athletes spread their fingers just a fraction, the water that's trapped between their fingers during the pull-throughs acts almost like a webbing and gives them an even stronger stroke. Seconds were shaved from the best times almost immediately after this new method was put into practice.

Athletes and coaches in all sports continue to discover effective performance variations, and bodybuilding practitioners are beginning to contribute their share of innovation. Part of the reason for these new advancements is that bodybuilding is finally gaining the respect it so rightfully deserves in the athletic community. Along with that respect comes more logical thought, experimentation and scientific analysis, the results of which are new, efficient training methods such as Positions of Flexion.

POF isn't the be-all and end-all of mass-training strategy. There are numerous other excellent programs available. I believe, however, that POF is one of the best and that, when properly applied, it has the potential to give anyone's bodybuilding training new life. Try the methods and routines in this book and see if you don't agree. Here's hoping that POF helps you set personal bodybuilding records of your own and achieve the physique you've always dreamed of.

John Balik
Publisher
*IRONMAN* Magazine

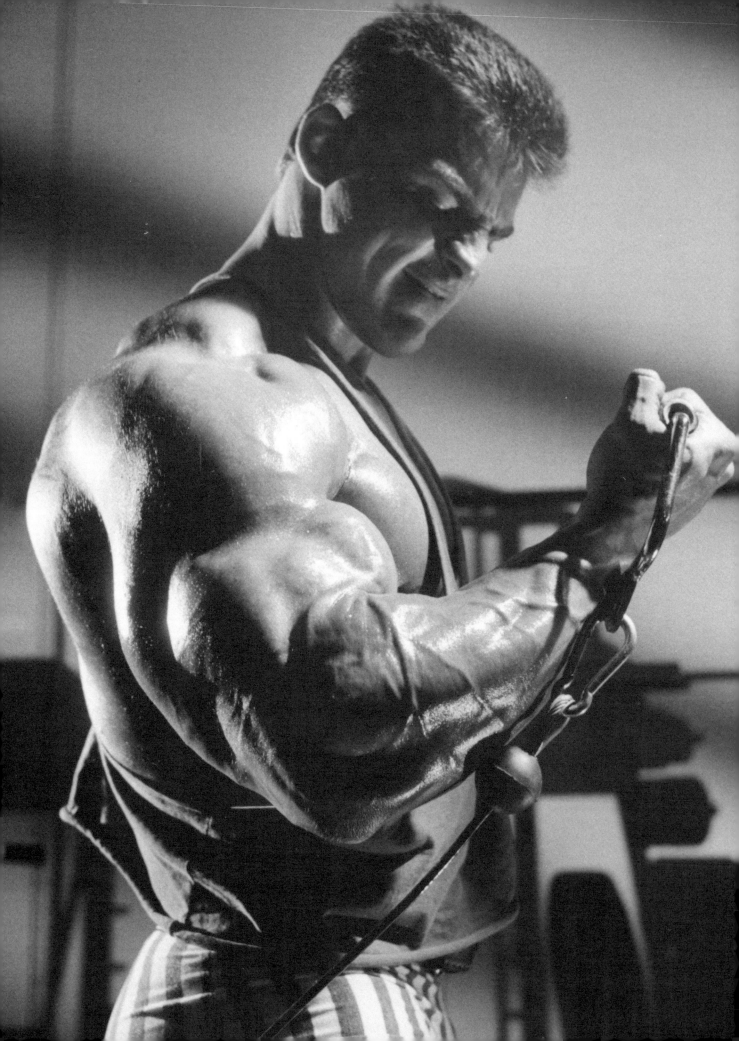

# INTRODUCTION

At no time in history has our species had such a massive breed of mortals in its midst. Today's bodybuilding champions are the most muscular humans ever to walk the planet, and compared to the average man, those gargantuan athletes look like completely different beings.

If you're a dedicated bodybuilder, you're no doubt trying to duplicate that type of extreme development. The question is, How? For most the course is obvious: Simply follow the champs' training protocols. Emulate those who have succeeded, and you, too, will succeed. But is that really the best way for you to achieve the most rapid mass gains possible? Not according to many experts who claim that the majority of the current physique champions train incorrectly and that they could have attained their amazing development faster and without the use of anabolic steroids if they'd trained more scientifically. A bold statement, to say the least, and one that you, the thinking bodybuilder, need to address as you zero in on the best way to build your own physique.

The first question you must ask yourself is, Should I follow the champions' lead, or do most of them actually train the wrong way? You'll no doubt come to the conclusion that because the champs have realized the type of radical development all bodybuilders crave, their training can't possibly be incorrect. And you'll be right. Their training isn't incorrect—at least not completely.

Look at any advanced bodybuilder's routine, and you'll see that it incorporates some form of multi-angular training, which means working every bodypart from more than one position in order to train each muscle in its entirety. This method, combined with high-intensity effort, is right on the money when it comes to stimulating full, complete development after the beginning and early-intermediate stages of training.

Having made this observation, we can't say that the champions train "wrong"; however, most of them do slow their gains significantly by training inefficiently and not as effectively as they could. Specifically, their routines involve a lot of angle overlap, which leads to inefficient sessions and overwork, and they often don't effectively train their muscles at the proper angles. This makes the second part of the experts' statement a fact. Most of the top stars could have come farther faster and without anabolic drugs if they had trained more scientifically.

First and foremost is the point that the typical advanced bodybuilder's routine is fraught with overlap. Take the average champion's quad routine, for example, which might include squats, leg presses and hack squats, among other exercises. Those three movements may appear to be the cornerstones of a great thigh workout, but if you analyze the action of each, you'll notice that they're very similar as far as training angles go—each works your thighs with an almost identical squatting-type movement. Many bodybuilders argue that the exercises hit the thigh muscles in slightly different ways, but the real fact is that the "slight" difference is so remote, it's not worth the extra effort and drain on your recovery ability.

Think about this inefficiency for a moment. If every bodybuilder's routine suffers from a similar overlap—and they almost all do—could overtraining be the primary reason that the majority of bodybuilders can't put on more than a few pounds of muscle a year? Absolutely. Most physique athletes overtrain to such a degree that they rarely allow their bodies to grow.

Consequently, your first step toward developing the ultimate mass-building strategy should be to eliminate the overlap in your routine. After that you must make sure you're training as effectively as possible by hitting the necessary angles—which means overhauling your current program and turning it into the most precise, high-intensity, multi-angular training strategy available. This involves targeting the muscles from three—and only three—angles, or positions: midrange, stretch and contracted.

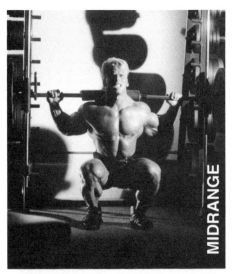

MIDRANGE

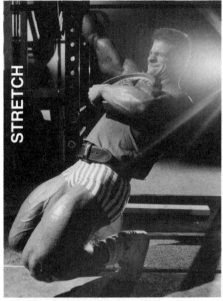

STRETCH

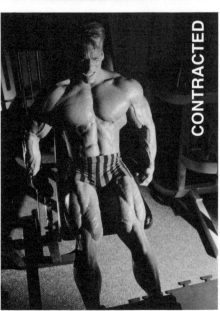

CONTRACTED

For example, let's say that you're using the thigh routine described above, and you decide to stick with squats, which cover the midrange position, as your first movement. As a result you cut out the hack squats and leg presses to eliminate the overlap. Then to effectively complete the multi-angular equation, you incorporate exercises that hit your thighs from the other two angles. You follow the squats with sissy squats, which give your quad routine a stretch component, and then finish off with leg extensions, which add a peak-contraction component. Now you've created an efficient multi-angular formula that effectively and completely works your quads by training them from three distinct positions—midrange, stretch and contracted. You completely fatigue your thighs without wasting precious energy—energy that your body will use for growth during the recovery process.

If you apply this three-position approach to each muscle group, you'll never use more than three exercises for any one bodypart, and many muscle groups will require even fewer because of the compound nature of certain movements. Also, if you train hard, you'll only need one to two sets of each exercise because of the laws of physiology and the precise, intense nature of this training method.

Here's a more general explanation of the three angles. The details of how these positions apply to each bodypart will follow in the forthcoming chapters.

•*Midrange.* You train this position with a multiple-joint, or compound, movement that works the muscle through more of a middle range without total peak contraction or stretch. Examples include squats or leg presses for the quads, overhead presses for the delts and bench presses for the pecs. Midrange movements often fall into the category of "big" exercises and tend to develop the bulk of the target muscle. Here are the criteria for most midrange exercises:

1) The target muscle doesn't reach its completely contracted state, which involves opposing resistance. With the bench press, for example, your arms never cross each other with opposite pulling forces, so your pecs don't reach this ultimate contracted position, as they do with, say, cable crossovers.

2) The target muscle doesn't receive a total stretch at any point during the range of motion. Although you may feel as if you're stretching your pecs at the bottom of a bench press, for example, they don't really achieve the type of stretch they're capable of, as they do with, say, dumbbell flyes.

3) Most midrange exercises work the target muscle group with the assistance of secondary muscles, which creates a synergistic effect. For instance, when you do squats, you work your quads, the target muscle group, with the help of your glutes and lower back. Because Mother Nature designed the human muscular system to function in

this manner—with the muscles working as a team—this synergistic effect allows you to stimulate the bulk of the target muscle with heavy weights as well as sufficiently warm it up for the more concentrated work to come in the next two positions.

•*Stretch.* In this position the target muscle reaches complete extension, where the fibers and fasciae, or fiber encasements, are in an extreme elongated state. As mentioned above, flyes satisfy this requirement for the pecs. Other stretch-position movements include pullovers for the lats, sissy squats for the quads, overhead extensions for the triceps and stiff-legged deadlifts for the hamstrings. Notice that at the bottom of each of these exercises you feel an uncomfortable pull on the target muscles, which allows you to take advantage of the prestretch phenomenon, an action that can help you involve more muscle fibers and create a more intense contraction in the target muscle. A good example of this prestretch reflex is what happens when a baseball player swings a bat; just before he swings, he abruptly forces the bat back to stretch the involved muscles. This quick twitch, also known as the myotatic reflex, gives him more power in his swing due to stronger neurological stimulation. You can get the same fiber-recruitment effect with stretch-position bodybuilding movements.

•*Contracted.* In this position the target muscle is placed in its ultimate peak-contracted, or flexed, state, which involves opposing resistance. In other words, when you reach the top of the movement, your limbs are in position for you to maximally contract the target muscle against resistance; that is, you have to fight to hold the weight in place, as with cable crossovers for the pecs. Because of this continuous resistance and the proper positioning of your limbs, you get an intense contraction. In order for you to get the best contraction possible, however, the muscle must be completely and thoroughly warmed up. This is why you usually work the contracted position last—to ensure that the muscle is warm. When you use a contracted-position exercise to finish off a bodypart workout, it contracts to its full capabilities against resistance through the entire range of motion. Other examples of contracted-position exercises include leg extensions for the quads, kickbacks for the triceps and leg curls for the hamstrings. Note that there is resistance in the top, or flexed, position of each of these exercises.

Midrange, stretch, contracted. By intensely training these three positions for every muscle group, you can completely work each bodypart with fewer sets, which leaves your recovery ability primed to produce explosive muscle growth. This is the basis of the Positions-of-Flexion (POF) training concept, a regimen that's exciting in its rationale and unparalleled in its ability to rapidly produce what you, the aspiring bodybuilder, crave, critical mass.

> **Midrange, stretch, contracted. By intensely training these three positions for every muscle group, you can completely work each bodypart with fewer sets, which leaves your recovery ability primed to produce explosive muscle growth.**

# 1
# CRITICAL
# CALVES

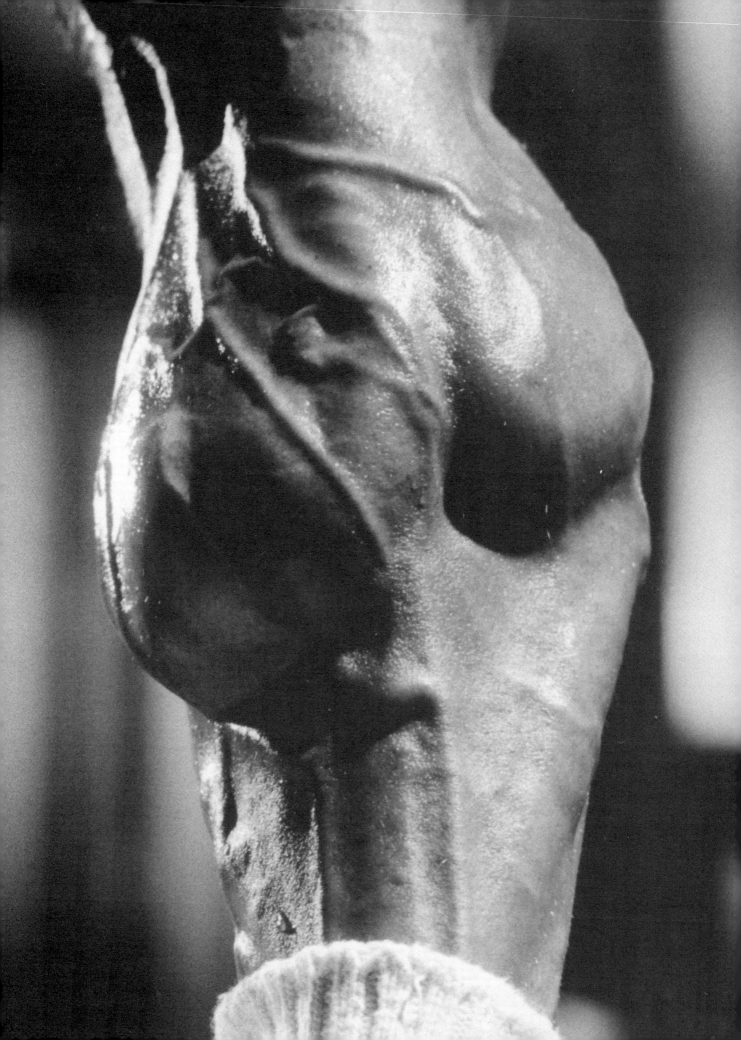

# A No-Bull Approach for Mass Below the Knees

Many bodybuilders make a big mistake that can lead to very small results when it comes to building calves. They look at the training of people who have mind-blowing lower legs, like former Mr. Olympia Chris Dickerson, for instance, and figure that he got those fabulous inverted hearts that are perched so regally below and behind his knees by training. There's a problem with such thinking, however. Some people are—like Chris—simply gifted in the calf area and will develop great lower legs from just walking around and other mild athletic activity. The fact is that Dickerson's calf development is almost totally the result of genetics.

The right way to learn about—or at least move toward—correct calf training is to look at the strategy of someone who has had to struggle to overcome a genetic weakness. In the case of calves, pro bodybuilder Robby Robinson is a prime example. At the beginning of Robby's career his lower legs seemed to be cursed. His high, diminutive calves knocked him down in every contest he entered. He didn't give up, though, and he eventually discovered an approach that blew up his calves to respectable proportions. Before long they were no longer a severe hindrance. In fact, they actually helped him win numerous amateur titles, including the '75 IFBB World Championships, and then go on to a successful pro bodybuilding career.

## Multi-Angular Calf Training

Robby's five-point plan to overcome his genetic lower-leg disadvantage was simple, as follows:

1) Hit the calves from all the required angles.

2) Do more reps per set.

3) Feel each repetition through the entire range of motion.

4) Don't neglect the soleus muscles.

5) Avoid overtraining the lower legs.

*Hit all the required angles.* Robby's multi-angular regimen consisted of doing numerous calf exercises, some sets with his toes pointed in, some with his toes pointed out and some with his toes pointed straight ahead. This shotgun approach isn't necessarily wrong, just inefficient, which means it can produce results, albeit slowly and with the ever-looming possibility of overtraining. In Robby's case it did eventually work, the reason being that by including so many movements and variations he did manage to hit his calves' primary positions of flexion. And when you train a muscle's three positions of flexion, you're in for some dramatic progress, especially if you avoid overtraining. The following are the positions of flexion for calf training:

*Midrange:* You work this position with toes-pointed leg curls—the hamstrings and calves work in tandem.

*Stretch:* You achieve this position at the bottom of a donkey calf raise—calves stretched off a high block, toes pointed slightly inward, knees locked and torso at a right angle to the legs. You should feel an uncomfortable pull on the gastrocnemius muscles in this position.

*Contracted:* You reach total contraction at the top of a standing calf raise—up on toes, torso and legs in line, or on the same plane, and toes pointed slightly outward. In this position you get peak contraction, which will finish off the gastrocs with all-out intensity.

So what Robby was doing, in effect, was correct; he was working all the positions of flexion by using a variety of exercises. If he had limited his exercise choice to one movement for each position, however, he would have eliminated the bouts of overtraining that he had to contend with on a regular basis, and he would have ensured full and complete development of his lower legs much more rapidly.

The above analysis of the positions of flexion for this muscle group indicates that the calf muscle, or gastrocnemius, requires only three exercises—if they're done correctly—to cover all the angles:

- toes-pointed leg curls
- donkey calf raises
- standing calf raises

Add an exercise like seated calf raises for your soleus muscles, which are broad, flat muscles that run down to your ankles under your gastrocs, and you have a routine that will pack your lower legs with mass.

Now that we've fine-tuned Robby's exercise choice, let's take a look at the other parts of his calf-massing plan.

*Higher reps.* The calf is one of the dens-

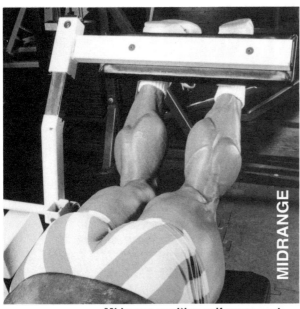

Midrange-position calf movement: toes-pointed leg curls.

Your foot angle enhances the position of flexion; it doesn't help you work the so-called inner or outer calves. For example, a toes-in stance on donkey calf raises (below) produces a better gastroc stretch than toes straight ahead or toes out, and a slight toes-out position on standing calf raises (below right) provides a better contraction.

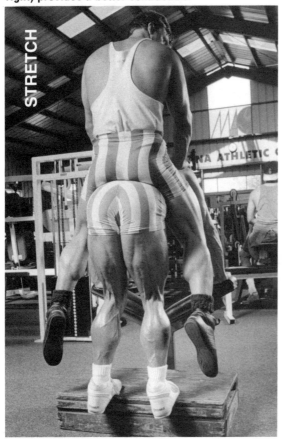

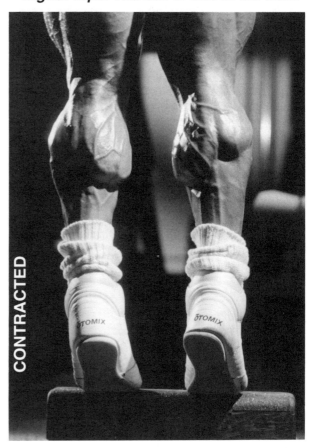

est muscle groups in the human muscular system. In other words, there are more fibers per square inch of calf muscle than there are in other muscles. This is why it takes a few more reps to get that painful-but-oh-so-productive growth burn from a set of calf raises—there are simply more muscle fibers to move the load and then fatigue. For best results work all gastrocnemius exercises with rep ranges of between 12 and 20.

*Feel.* As with any muscle group you must put your mind into the muscle and avoid bouncing and/or throwing the weight. Rep speed is also important. Three seconds up and three seconds down is just about right. This slightly exaggerated slowness—you use a two-seconds-up, two-seconds-down rep cadence for other muscle groups—is a must for complete calf development because it enables you to get in touch with the muscle during each contraction.

Another aspect that should be exaggerated is the range of motion. Many trainees don't go all the way up or all the way down, and then they wonder why their calves don't respond. You've probably seen these individuals. Every gym has at least one guy with pipe-cleaner lower legs who pumps out his calf raises while moving about three inches per rep. It doesn't matter how many sets of partial calf raises you do, your calves will never look complete until you work them from total stretch to total contraction.

*Soleus.* Developing this muscle not only gives the gastrocs a fuller appearance, but it also makes the area between the gastrocs and the ankle meatier. Trainees who have high calves should never neglect soleus work. A developed soleus will give the illusion of a lower gastrocnemius and help diffuse a glaring high-calf appearance, the very reason you should hit your soleus muscles hard.

As mentioned above, the best exercise for soleus development is seated calf raises. Be sure that your lower legs are at 90 degree angles to your thighs on this movement—no more, no less. This is the optimal position for soleus involvement and will ensure that the target muscles get an intense contraction. The seated calf raise is a contracted-position movement for the soleus. You work the soleus' midrange position with toes-pointed leg curls and its stretch position with donkey calf raises, both of which perform the same functions for the gastrocs. Therefore, you only have to add the one exercise for the soleus.

*Overtraining.* Walking, climbing in and out of cars and getting up from chairs all

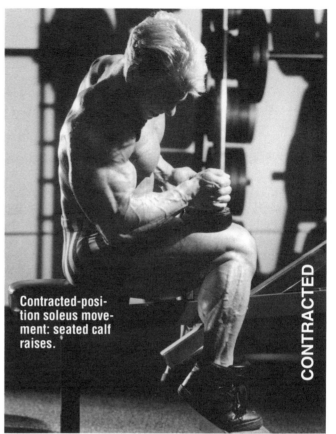

Contracted-position soleus movement: seated calf raises.

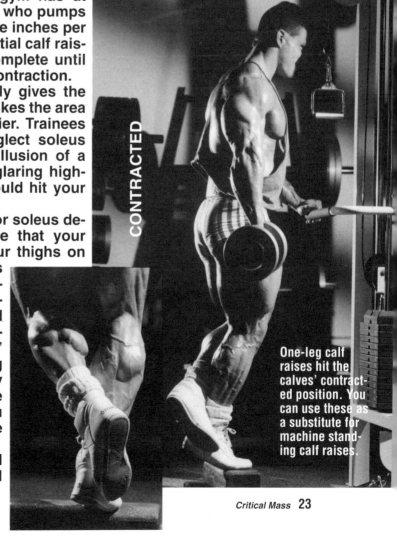

One-leg calf raises hit the calves' contracted position. You can use these as a substitute for machine standing calf raises.

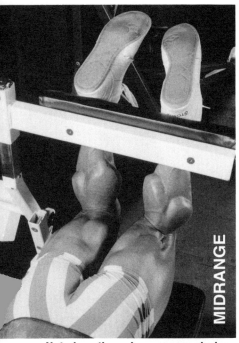

Note how the calves engage during toes-pointed leg curls. This is a midrange movement for the calves.

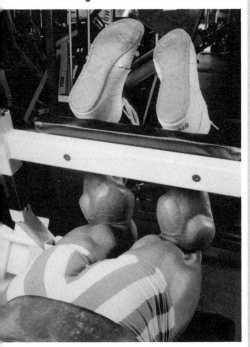

have an effect on the calves, but unless you're a mail carrier or a professional dancer or you have some other leg-oriented job, your calves really don't receive much work from such low-intensity, low-duration daily activity. Nevertheless, the calves are as susceptible to the perils of overtraining as any other muscle group. Consequently, there's no reason ever to do more than nine sets for your calves, including the soleus, if you work all of your sets hard, and it's usually better to do even fewer. Also, you should never train your calves more than three times per week—and twice per week is preferable.

Here's an example of a POF calf routine that will work wonders on practically anyone's lower legs:

### POF Calf Routine

**Gastrocnemius**

*Midrange:*
Toes-pointed leg curls   1-2 x 12-20
(*Don't pause at the top or bottom.*)

*Stretch:*
Donkey calf raises
   or leg press calf raises   2 x 12-20
(*Point your toes in slightly for maximum stretch, and at the bottom, or point of stretch, use a quick twitch for a more intense contraction.*)

*Contracted:*
Standing calf raises
   or hack machine
   calf raises   2 x 12-20
(*Point your toes out slightly and pause at the top of each rep for two to three seconds for maximum contraction.*)

**Soleus**

*Contracted\*:*
Seated calf raises   2 x 12-20
(*Point your toes straight ahead and pause for two to three seconds at the top of each rep.*)

\*You work the soleus muscles' midrange position during the toes-pointed leg curls and the stretch position with donkey calf raises, so there's no need to specifically target these positions.

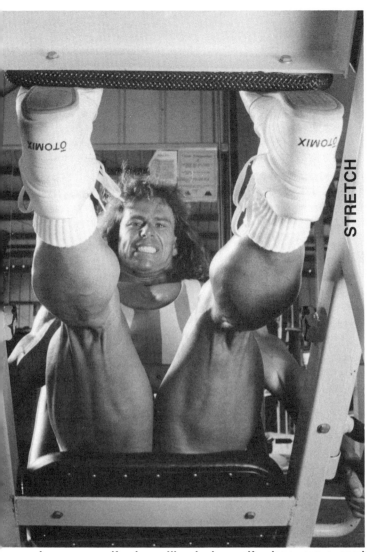
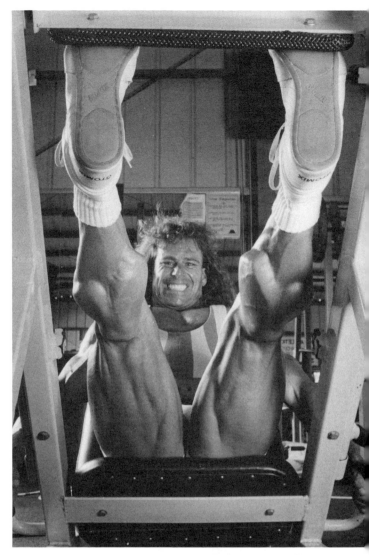
STRETCH

Leg press calf raises, like donkey calf raises, are a good stretch-position exercise for the calves. Note that you should keep your toes pointed slightly inward.

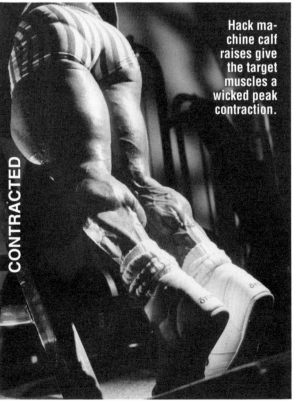
CONTRACTED

Hack machine calf raises give the target muscles a wicked peak contraction.

Eight sets may not look like much on paper, but if you treat every set as if it's the last one of your life, you'll get all the intensity you need for rapid mass gains. Research has substantiated the fact that the key to muscle growth is intensity of effort, so if you take every set other than warmups to where you can't get another out, you'll seldom need more than one or two sets for any exercise because you completely fatigue the muscle in the position you're working. After that it's time to move on to the next position.

No matter what angle you're using, the target muscles work according to what's called the all-or-nothing principle—either a muscle fiber contracts, or it does no work at all. For example, when you do machine calf raises, on your first rep your brain signals the muscle that it needs, say, 100 fibers to move the load. All of the 100 fibers contract completely. On the next rep those 100 fibers again contract completely, but because they're now weaker, more fibers must be recruited to move the load. Let's say you need 10 extra

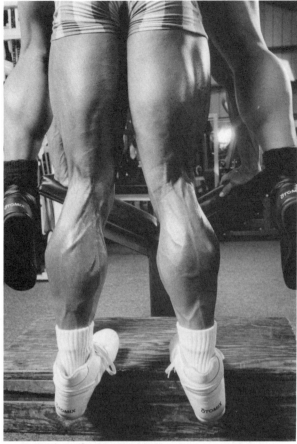

A quick twitch in the bottom, stretch position of the donkey calf raise will help you involve more muscle fibers.

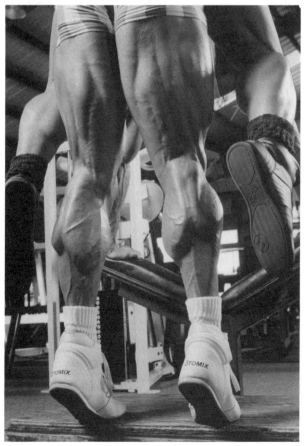

fibers. Now you have 110 fibers (100 + 10) contracting maximally. The process continues until the end of the set, and by your last rep you're contracting a very high percentage of the fibers in the target muscle group. [Note that there are always fibers left in reserve, and techniques such as prestretch can force more of them to work rather than rest.] Because of the all-or-nothing principle, one set will completely fatigue the muscle in a given position if you work the set to failure. This is why you can't do as many reps on a second set with the same weight—the fibers have already been depleted.

Some people find it difficult to generate enough intensity with one set, so they may need two. If you feel as if you've intensely contracted the target muscle with one set, however, move on to the next exercise. You'll conserve that much more recovery ability for growth. As Dorian Yates, the '92 and '93 Mr. Olympia put it, "I don't believe in doing the traditional 15 to 20 sets per bodypart. That's too much work. I'll do one or two sets per exercise. If you haven't done the job by then, it's not going to happen."

As you can see, the above routine works the calves from all angles and really gets the nutrient-rich blood pumping. If you have stubborn calves, give this no-bull POF approach a try and watch in amazement as your calves mature into full-grown heifers.

### Exercise Descriptions

*Toes-pointed leg curls.* Perform leg curls but keep your toes pointed away from your shins throughout the set. This will force your calves and hamstrings to work together to get the weight up.

*Donkey calf raises.* Bend at the waist, with your torso 90 degrees to your thighs, and rest your forearms on a table, high bench or racked barbell. Elevate the balls of your feet on a calf block, and have your training partner sit on your hips. Do calf raises with your toes pointing slightly inward until failure. Although it's important to feel the stretch, don't hold at the bottom of the rep. You want to take advantage of the prestretch phenomenon, so as soon as you reach the lowest position, reverse the movement and fire out another rep. The key to getting the most out of stretch-position exercises is to eliminate the pause at the point of stretch.

*Standing calf raises.* Adjust the shoulder pads so that you feel resistance in your lowest position, place the pin in the weight stack and get comfortable under the pads. With your toes pointing slightly outward, lift the weight and drive up until you reach full calf contraction. Hold for a count of two and then lower slowly. It's important to get a good flex at the top of any contracted-position exercise. Also, keep your knees locked throughout the movement to keep the soleus out of the action.

*Seated calf raises.* Load the machine, then sit down and adjust the height until your knees are bent at 90 degree angles when they're under the pads and the balls of your feet are on the footpads. Get in position and release the weight. Stretch down as far as you can go and then push the weight up until you're on your toes. Hold for a count of two, then slowly lower back to the bottom and repeat.

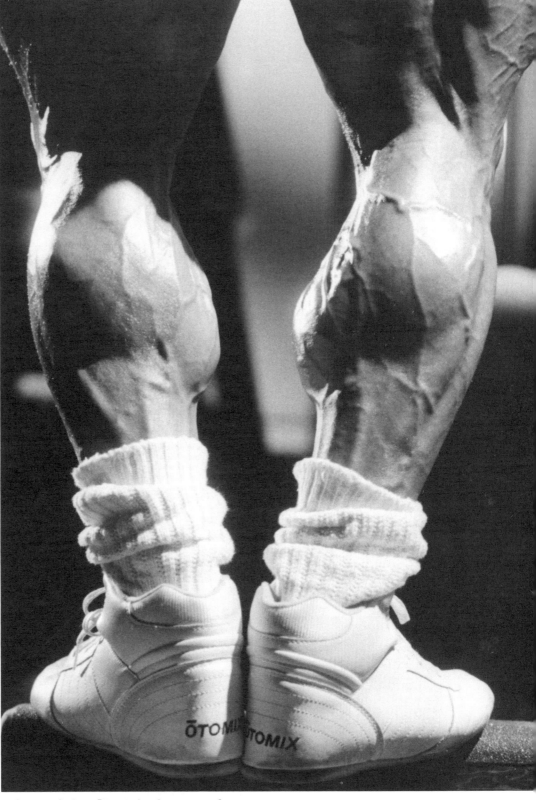

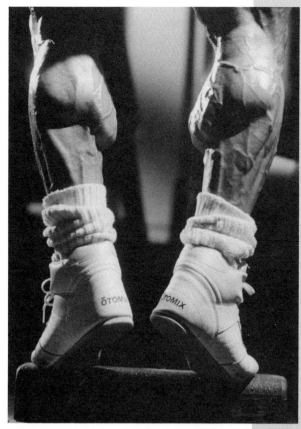

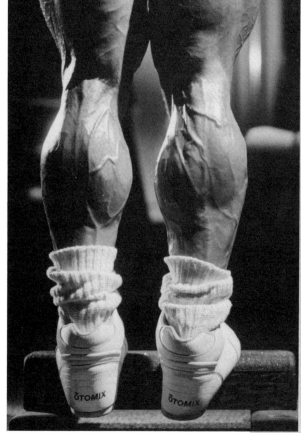

## Critical Calf Q & A

*Q: Shouldn't I use all the various foot positions—toes in, toes out and toes straight ahead—for each calf exercise if I want total development?*

*A:* The different foot positions do have an effect on calf development but only as they relate to the positions of flexion. In other words, it's working each muscle from the three positions of flexion that gives the calves their full, complete look, and foot angle simply makes the work in each position more effective. Notice that in order for you to get into the maximum stretch position, your torso must be at 90 degrees to your thighs, your heels below your toes and your toes pointing slightly inward, as they are for toes-in donkey calf raises; in order for you to reach the total contracted position, your torso and thighs must be on the same plane, your heels above your toes and your toes pointing slightly outward, as they are for toes-out standing calf raises. So, in effect, you're working the toes-in position with donkey calf raises and the toes-out position with standing calf raises, but you do this only to enhance the stretch and contraction, respectively, not in a random shotgun fashion, or, as many trainees believe, to work your so-called inner and outer calves.

*Q: Won't the regular leg curls that I do in my thigh routine work the calves' midrange position enough that I don't have to do the toes-pointed leg curls?*

*A:* Although your calves will get some midrange work from regular leg curls, it's not enough to eliminate the need for including the toes-pointed variety in your calf routine. Remember, when you do regular leg curls, you focus on the hamstrings, and if you do them with your toes flexed toward your shins, as you should when training hams, then you remove a lot of the stress from the calves and place it directly on the hams. Conversely, when you do a leg curl with your toes pointed, your calves are more directly involved in the movement. Do at least one set of toes-pointed leg curls to ensure that your calves get enough midrange work.

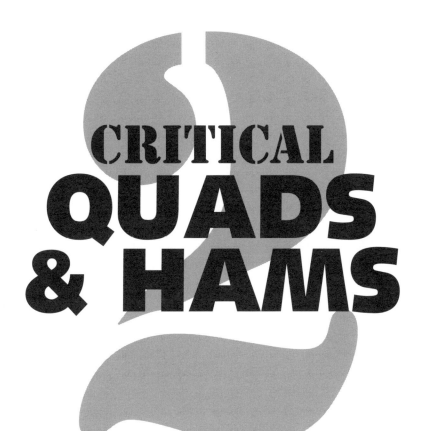

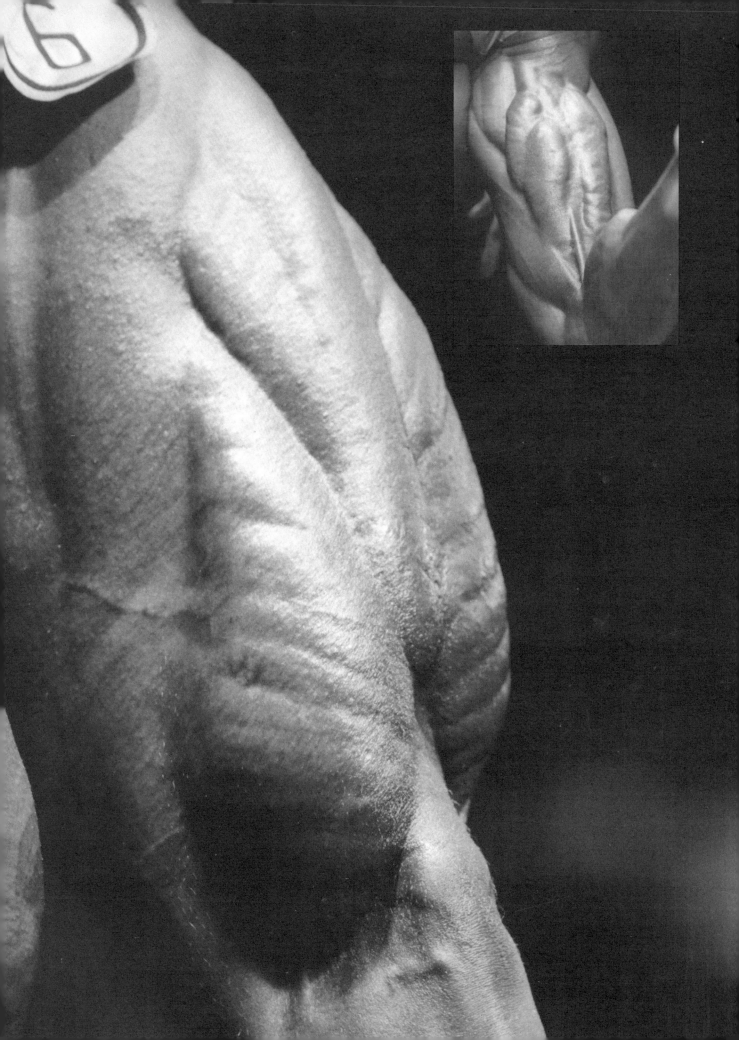

# Build Tree-Trunk-Size Thighs

An extraordinarily developed pair of thighs is a wonder to behold—a world-class sprinter's quads and hamstrings contracting and relaxing almost quicker than the eye can focus, a cyclist's well-muscled legs pumping the pedals like the pistons in a V-8 and, of course, a bodybuilder's thick, striated quadriceps jumping and separating with each lock of his knee.

Without a doubt, the competitive bodybuilder sports the most impressively developed thighs of all athletes and rightly so. The bodybuilder must have outlandish size and proportion in all muscle groups to excel on the posing dais—the kind of development that causes even the most massive athletes in other sports to stare in amazement.

The bodybuilder's extraordinary development occurs because of the nature of the activity—concentrated training effort tailored specifically to build muscle mass. The development that other athletes acquire is merely a side effect of their activities, while the bodybuilder blasts each bodypart into submission *in order to grow larger and stronger*. Muscle growth is the desired end result, not just an incidental benefit. It's the bodybuilder's obsession.

As with any obsession, however, the quest for size can be overdone to the point of irrational behavior, which in the bodybuilder's case often translates into gain-halting overtraining, especially when a large bodypart like the thighs is taxing recovery ability.

## Overlap and Overtraining

To achieve extreme development, advanced bodybuilders attempt to work each muscle group from every possible angle, and the thighs are no exception. They often include leg presses, squats, hack squats, sissy squats, leg extensions, leg curls, stiff-legged deadlifts and one-leg leg curls all in the same routine, and some of those every-exercise-in-the-book programs could send a full-grown gorilla to the intensive care unit.

Bodybuilders view this approach as necessary for complete development. The logic is simple enough. Inordinate size gains in the late-intermediate-to-advanced levels of training require a multiangular attack in order to hit all the muscle fibers, which means countless exercises for the thighs and hamstrings—or does it?

If you analyze this type of all-encompassing thigh workout with a logical eye, you'll see the wasted effort. Squats and leg presses, for example, work the quads in relatively the same manner, an unnecessary overlap that's highly inefficient and can cause overtraining. The average lifter can actually lose muscle on such a program.

Training more efficiently means using the least amount of exercise necessary in order to conserve your recovery ability while still getting total growth stimulation. You want to train your muscles completely and leave plenty of your body's reserves intact, which enhances the mass-building processes. All bodybuilders should be focused on efficiency and ultimate effectiveness in the gym if they want to have enough energy left for the most rapid muscle growth possible, a.k.a. critical mass.

## POF Thigh Strategy

To reiterate, the Positions-of-Flexion training philosophy states that each muscle or muscle group has only three positions at which it must be trained for total development—midrange, stretch and contracted. Let's take the quadriceps and hamstrings and analyze each group's positions of flexion.

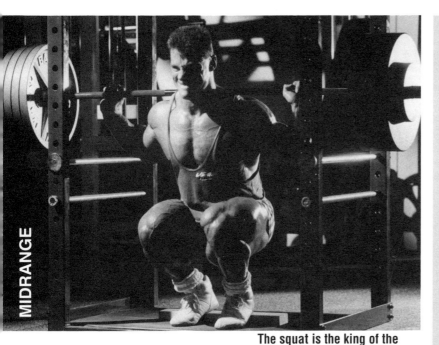

MIDRANGE

The squat is the king of the midrange-quad movements. Your glutes and lower back provide synergy for your quads, which are the prime movers in this exercise.

## Quads

*Midrange:* Squatting or leg press movements take care of this position. Notice that there's no full stretch or peak contraction of the target muscles during these exercises and that the hips and hamstrings act in tandem with the quads to move the weight.

*Stretch:* The bottom of a sissy squat—torso and thighs on the same plane, calves almost flush against the hamstrings—places the quads in a full stretch.

*Contracted:* The top of a leg extension—torso and thighs at a right angle, lower legs extended and knees locked—peak-contracts the quads. Note that there's resistance in the top position.

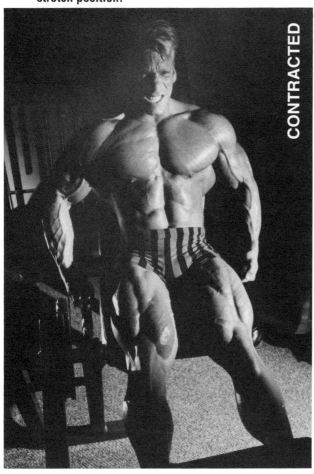

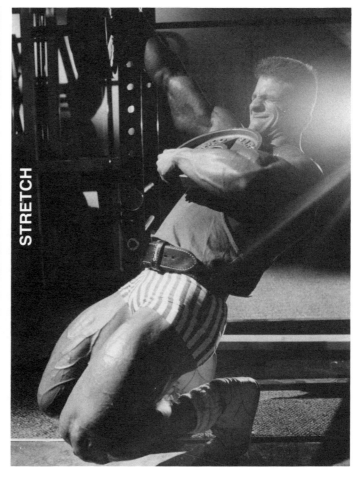

Leg extensions work the quads' contracted position, while sissy squats (right) take care of the stretch position.

CONTRACTED

STRETCH

## Hamstrings

*Midrange:* The middle-to-top portion of a stiff-legged deadlift or squat works this position.

*Stretch:* The bottom of a stiff-legged deadlift puts the hamstrings in a full stretch.

*Contracted:* The top of a leg curl—torso and thighs on the same plane, calves almost flush against the hamstrings and feet flexed toward the shins—provides peak contraction for the hams. Note once again that there's resistance in the top position.

By analyzing the three positions, you can see that the quadriceps, or frontal thighs, require three movements, while the hamstrings only require two to work all three positions of flexion. A good, growth-inducing POF thigh routine would look like the following. To promote maximum efficiency, this regimen also includes the lower back. You work your lower back after thighs and hamstrings to take advantage of the fact that you already worked that bodypart's midrange and stretch positions with stiff-legged deadlifts.

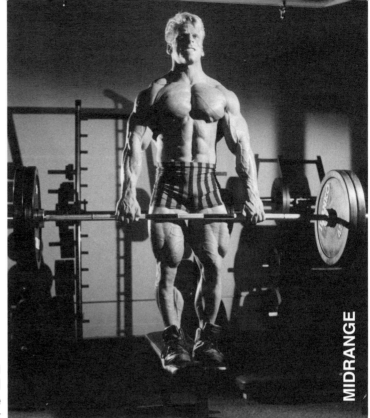

The top one-third of the stiff-legged deadlift works the hamstring's midrange position, while the bottom works the stretch position.

The top of a leg curl rep provides peak contraction for the hamstrings, which makes leg curls a contracted-position movement.

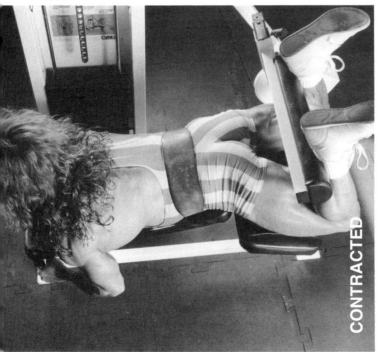

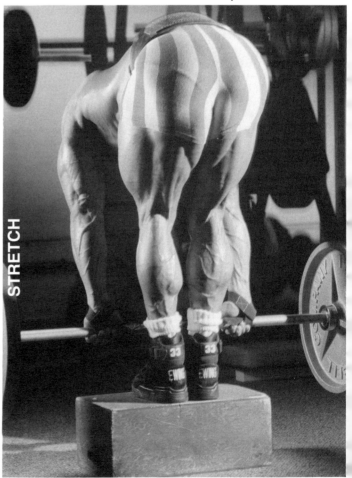

Critical Mass 33

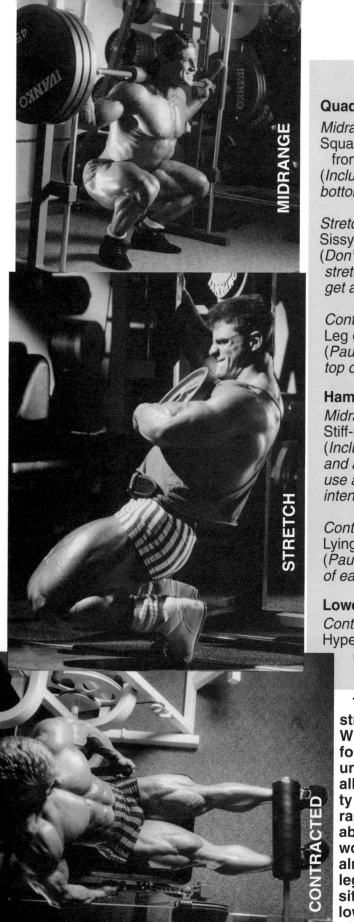

## POF Thigh & Lower-Back Routine

### Quads

*Midrange:*
Squats, leg presses,
 front squats or Smith machine squats   2 x 8-12
(*Include little or no pause at the top or bottom.*)

*Stretch:*
Sissy squats   2 x 8-12
(*Don't pause at the bottom, or point of stretch, but instead use a quick twitch to get a more intense contraction.*)

*Contracted:*
Leg extensions   1-2 x 8-12
(*Pause for two to three seconds at the top of each rep for peak contraction.*)

### Hams

*Midrange & Stretch:*
Stiff-legged deadlifts   2 x 8-12
(*Include little or no pause at the top, and at the bottom, or point of stretch, use a quick twitch to get a more intense contraction.*)

*Contracted:*
Lying or standing leg curls   1-2 x 8-12
(*Pause for two to three seconds at the top of each rep for peak contraction.*)

### Lower Back

*Contracted:*
Hyperextensions   2 x 8-12
 (*Pause for two to three seconds at the top of each rep for peak contraction.*)

That's six sets for quads, four sets for hamstrings and two sets to finish off the lower back. While these set totals may seem low, if you perform each set to momentary muscular failure—until you can't get another rep—as you should for all bodyparts and periodically incorporate intensity techniques, such as forced reps, you'll get full, rapid growth without wasting precious recovery ability. Remember, there's no overlap as far as working the various angles is concerned. There's almost no wasted effort. In the case of the stiff-legged deadlift, one exercise works two of the positions of flexion on both the hamstrings and the lower back, which makes the routine even more efficient.

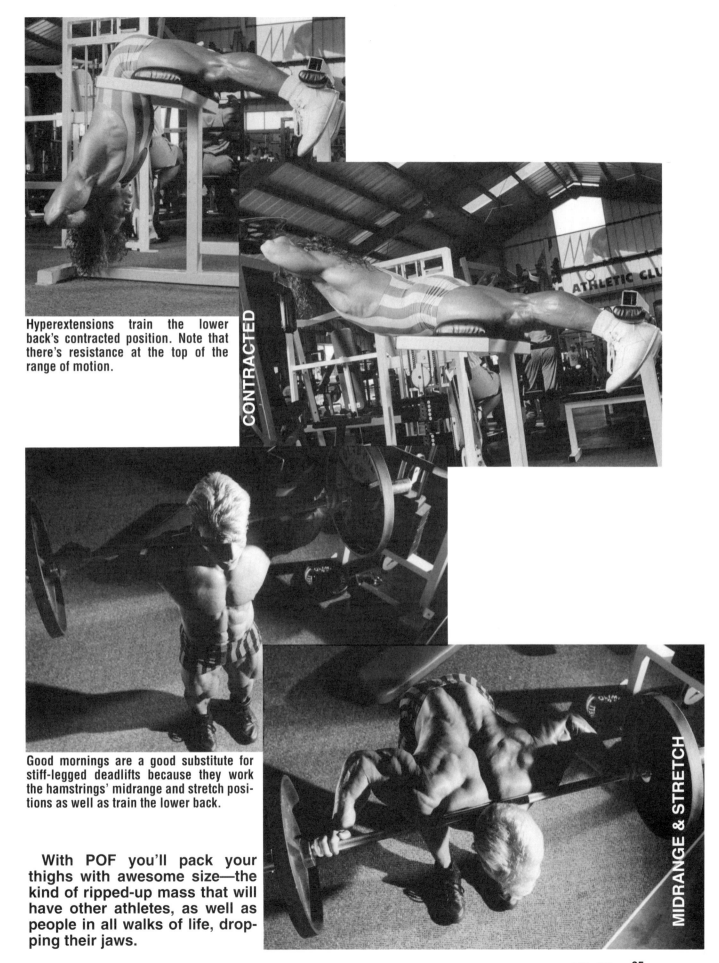

Hyperextensions train the lower back's contracted position. Note that there's resistance at the top of the range of motion.

CONTRACTED

Good mornings are a good substitute for stiff-legged deadlifts because they work the hamstrings' midrange and stretch positions as well as train the lower back.

With POF you'll pack your thighs with awesome size—the kind of ripped-up mass that will have other athletes, as well as people in all walks of life, dropping their jaws.

MIDRANGE & STRETCH

## Exercise Descriptions

*Squats.* Take a loaded barbell off a rack and place it across your shoulders. Back away from the rack, take a comfortable stance and squat until your thighs are just below parallel to the floor. You may want to put a two-by-four-inch board under your heels for better form and balance. Also, be sure to look straight ahead throughout the movement to prevent your lower back from arching, and keep your torso as upright as possible to maximize thigh involvement. Repeat.

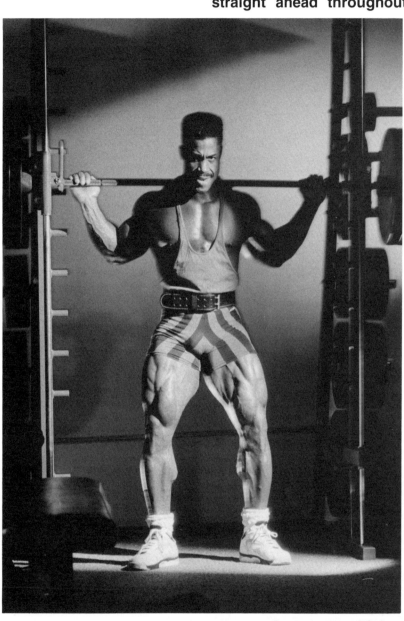

*Sissy squats.* Hold onto an upright with one hand and bend your knees while keeping your thighs and torso in the same plane—don't bend at the waist. Lean back as far as possible as you squat (at the bottom you'll be in position to do the limbo). Your knees will move forward, and you'll feel a tremendous stretch in your thighs when you get to the bottom. Don't pause there, however. You want to take advantage of the prestretch phenomenon, so as soon as you reach the bottom, reverse direction and begin another rep—a quick twitch to recruit more muscle fibers. Without prestretch you fatigue the majority of the fibers in this position, as dictated by the all-or-none principle; with it you get closer to fatiguing all of the fibers, as fewer are left in reserve at the end of the set. As you gain strength on sissy squats, hold a barbell plate on your chest. Once that becomes too light, you can improvise and do them on a Smith machine, with the bar on your chest.

*Leg extensions.* Load a leg extension machine, sit down and hook your feet under the roller pads. With your torso at a 90 degree angle to your thighs, raise, or extend, your lower legs until your quadriceps contract. Hold this position for a count of two while squeezing your quads hard. This is a contracted-position movement, so emphasize the top.

*Stiff-legged deadlifts on a bench.* Load a bar on a pair of bench uprights, stand on the bench, lift the bar and take a step back. Holding the bar at arm's length in front of your thighs, slowly bend at the waist while keeping the bar close to your legs. When the bar is a few inches from hitting the bench, reverse direction for that important prestretch and slowly pull your torso back to the upright position. The safest way to perform this exercise is with your back flat at all times—no rounding. This emphasizes the hamstrings over the lower back, however, as the lower back never reaches its stretch position. To emphasize the lower back, slightly round your back during deadlifts. Try using the slightly rounded position on your first set and keeping your back flat on your second. This strategy enables you to target your lower back on one intense set and your hamstrings on the other. If you're prone to lower-back aches and pains, skip the rounded-back version, as it places more stress on the spine.

*Leg curls.* Load the leg curl apparatus, lie facedown on the machine and position the backs of your lower legs under the roller pads. Curl your lower legs up, keeping your feet flexed toward your shins, until the pads touch your buttocks. Hold for a count of two, lower and repeat.

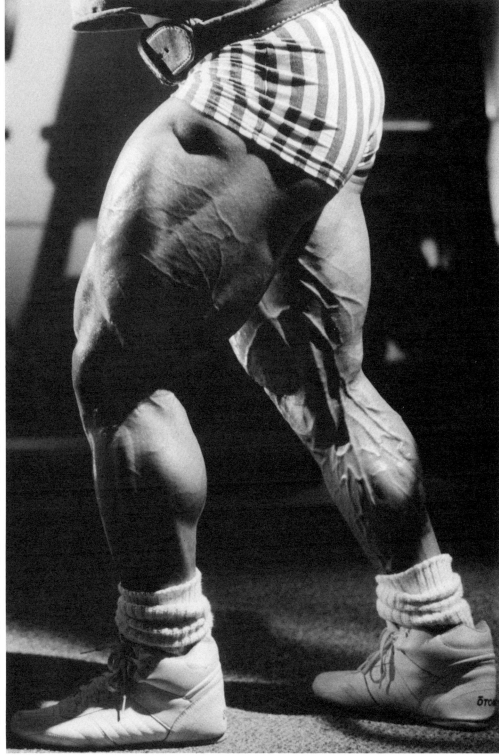

*Hyperextensions.* Position yourself on a hyperextension bench and lower your torso until it's at a right angle to your legs. Raise your torso until it's slightly above parallel to the floor, hold for a count of two—remember, this is a contracted-position movement—and then slowly lower back to the bottom. As soon as your torso and legs hit that right angle, begin another rep.

## Critical Quads and Hams Q & A

*Q: Is the hack squat on a machine a midrange-, stretch- or contracted-position exercise?*

*A:* Regular hack squats fall into the midrange category. They're almost identical to regular barbell squats except the hack machine eliminates a lot of lower-back involvement. On some hack machines, however, you can turn them into a stretch-position exercise by keeping your hips out away from the back pad. With this technique the hack squat becomes a sissy hack squat and allows you to take advantage of the prestretch phenomenon, which will give you a more powerful muscular contraction.

*Q: Why two sets? Can't I get all I need from one?*

*A:* Yes and no. As discussed in Chapter 1, the all-or-nothing principle of muscle contraction does indicate that one set will fatigue almost all of the muscle fibers in one position; however, at the end of a set there are still some fresh fibers. Forced reps will help recruit these fresh fibers, or you can do one more set, which will give you a different recruitment pattern and call those leftover fresh fibers into play early on.

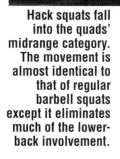

Hack squats fall into the quads' midrange category. The movement is almost identical to that of regular barbell squats except it eliminates much of the lower-back involvement.

Another reason to use two sets is that different foot positions and hand positions can change leverages and take certain muscle groups out of the movement on many exercises. For example, when you do squats with your feet shoulder width apart, you involve the quadriceps as well as the adductors, or inner thighs, and glutes. If on your next set you put your feet closer together, you essentially take the adductors out of the movement. In other words, you get less synergy—or less help from surrounding muscles—and you put more stress directly on the quads and glutes.

So in answer to your question, if you do one set to failure plus forced reps, move on, but if you do one set without forced reps, do another set to positive failure to hit all of the available fibers. You may also want to use a slightly different foot or hand placement on this second set for more or less of a direct hit on the target muscle.

Remember that synergy—the muscles working as a team—is important during midrange movements, so you should go for as much teamwork as possible on these exercises for maximum midrange benefit.

Also, never make drastic changes in foot or hand placement, as you'll set yourself up for an injury. If you use an extremely wide grip on any type of upper-body pressing, for example, you can damage your shoulder joints, and wide-stance squats can injure hip and knee joints. Use only slight alterations when it comes to grip and stance widths.

*Q: Are lunges a good midrange thigh exercise?*

*A:* Yes, but you have to do them correctly to get the full thigh-building potential. Stand with your feet about shoulder width apart with a loaded bar across your shoulders. Step forward and slightly to the side with your right leg, slowly bending both knees until your left knee touches the floor and your right is out over your toes. The angle at your right knee should be less than 45 degrees in this low position. Without any momentum—and this is very important—push back up out of the lunge with your right leg, and when your legs are straight or almost straight step back into the starting position and repeat with your left leg. You can also do this one leg at a time instead of alternating. When you come up out of the lunge on your right leg, don't step back but rather continue doing reps with that leg. When you finish the set, rest and repeat with your left leg. Another alternative that's a favorite of six-time Ms. Olympia Cory Everson is to step back with the nonworking leg instead of forward with the working leg. This style may help you maintain your balance. Some people find that lunges hurt their knees. If you're one of them, avoid this movement.

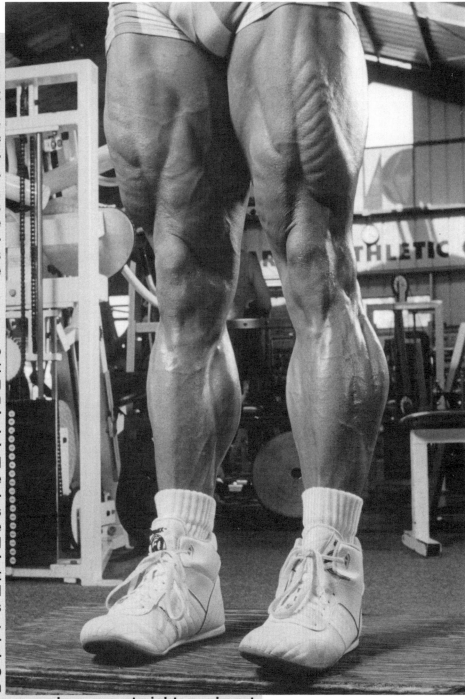

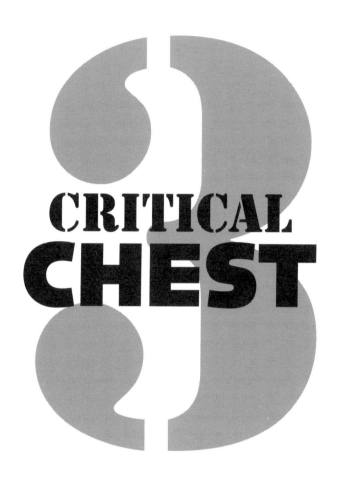

# CRITICAL CHEST

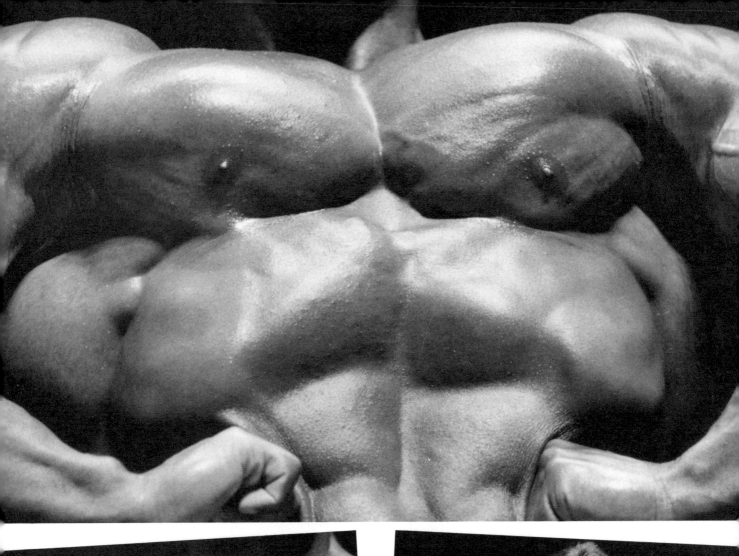
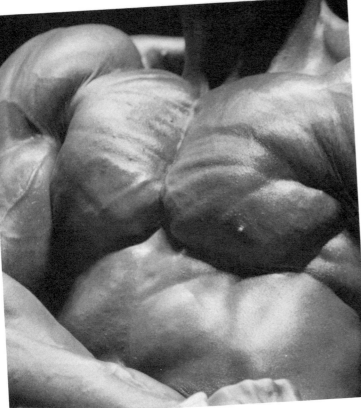
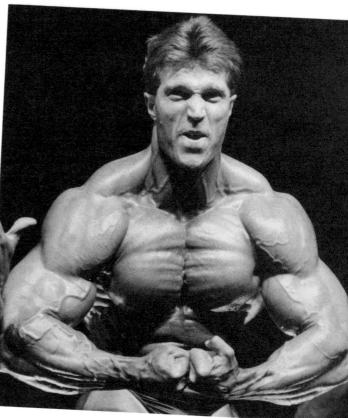

# The Quest for Pec Perfection

It was spring break, and all the hotel guests were out by the pool, basking in the warm midday sun. College students from across the country had come to Texas' South Padre Island for a one-week hiatus, but the trials and tribulations of academia were still the predominant topic of conversation—until he arrived, that is.

Clad in baggy bright orange beach jams, which couldn't begin to hide his massive quads and hams, and a white torso-hugging York Barbell Club T-shirt, this man had obviously been hitting the iron hard. The loud conversations around the pool turned to whispers as he pulled up a lounge chair, spread his towel and began peeling off his shirt, every one of his movements a veritable lesson in muscular anatomy.

As his shirt came off and his arms came down from above his head, the poolside populace let out an astonished gasp. And for good reason. The man was a work of art, every muscle developed in perfect harmony with every other.

One coed who was sitting nearby turned to her friend and said, "The scenery just improved 100 percent. Look at that chest."

In fact, it was a perfect chest—with deep lines etching the lower portions from delt to sternum, a split separating the upper and lower pecs that jumped into view every time he moved his arms and a fireworks display of striations that exploded all the way up to his clavicles. What was really amazing was how his chest development was so perfectly balanced—high, full pecs that brought Steve Reeves to mind.

So who was this guy? Was he Mr. America or Mr. Universe, or had the gods sent him down from the heavens to show the mere mortals how inferior their own physiques were? No one ever found out. You see, no self-respecting male was going to put his body into comparison range of this Adonis just to ask him a few questions. That would have been like giving the women around the pool the choice between T-bone steak and a corn dog.

### The Specs for Perfect Pecs

Just what makes a perfect pair of pecs? Fullness and shape are definitely important. High, full pectorals have been the desire of almost everyone who has ever reclined on an exercise bench. Shawn Ray, Bob Paris and Samir Bannout are just a few examples of physique stars who have near-perfect chests. When bodybuilders have well-proportioned pecs, as these men do, they radiate power even in street clothes. And talk about confidence. A great upper torso gives a lifter that chest-held-high look that commands respect in any situation.

To attain perfect pecs you must avoid the cross-your-heart pec preponderance and, on the opposite end of the spectrum, the flat-chested, where's-the-beef look. If you want balanced development, what you need, plain and simple, is a logical, straightforward workout strategy.

### POF Pec Attack

Whether your problem is too much or too little in the way of chest development, you need a balanced, rational training approach that includes some kinesiology—a game plan that will give your pecs dramatic shape and size in proper proportions and in the shortest time possible. The POF approach is just such a strategy.

To reiterate, POF chucks the shotgun method of bodypart training—working each muscle with an overabundance of exercise to "hit as many angles as possible"—and instead uses a more pragmatic approach to push each bodypart to spectacular levels of development. Your first step in creating the ultimate pec program is to observe the muscle itself. If you've

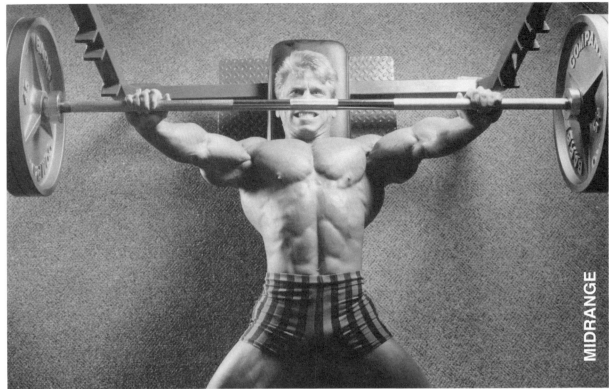

The bench press is the most popular midrange movement for the lower pecs.

been bodybuilding for any length of time, you know that the pectorals each have an upper and a lower segment—the pectoralis minor and pectoralis major, respectively. Technically, the pecs major cover the entire chest area, and the pecs minor lie under the upper portions of the pecs major. For complete development, however, you must treat the upper and lower pecs as two separate entities, as follows:

Decline cable flyes allow you to train two low-pec positions—stretch and contracted—with one movement.

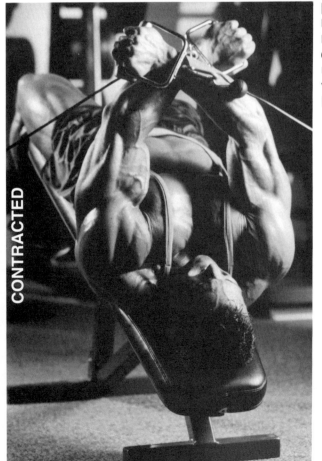

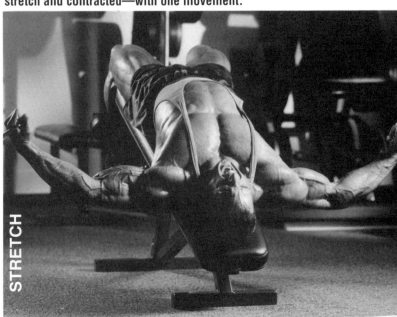

44  *Critical Mass*

#### Upper pecs

*Midrange:* Any incline pressing movement works the midrange position. The triceps and front delts help the upper pecs move the weight.

*Stretch:* The bottom of an incline flye puts the upper pecs into a complete stretch position.

*Contracted:* You reach peak contraction when your arms are extended and crossed over your upper chest with resistance in this position, as in the top of an incline cable flye.

#### Lower pecs

*Midrange:* Any flat or decline pressing movement hits this position. The triceps and front delts help your pecs major move the resistance.

*Stretch:* The bottom of a decline flye—elbows back behind the torso, arms wide—completely stretches the lower pecs.

*Contracted:* You reach total peak contraction when your arms are extended and crossed at midforearm below your lower chest, as in a standard cable crossover.

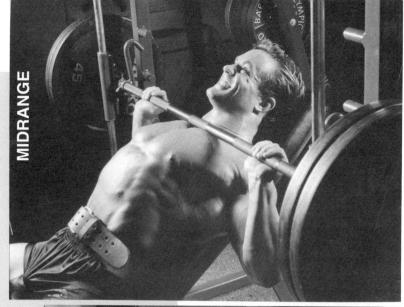

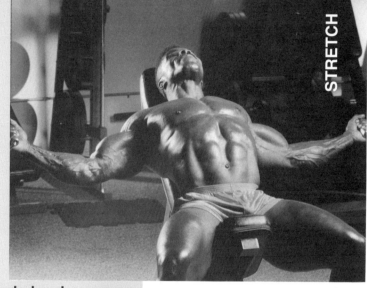

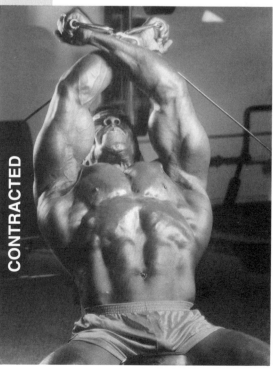

After reading through this analysis, you might be thinking, "Wait a minute. Six exercises? I thought this was going to be an efficient chest routine!" Fortunately, one movement often takes care of two of the positions of flexion, as you saw in Chapter 2 with the deadlift, which works the hamstrings' midrange and stretch positions. Both pec areas qualify for the two-in-one scenario: Incline cable flyes work the upper pecs' stretch and contracted positions, while flat or decline cable flyes or cable crossovers hit the lower pecs' stretch and contracted positions. That gives you a total of two exercises for the upper chest and two for the lower. Here's an example of a simple, solid POF pec routine:

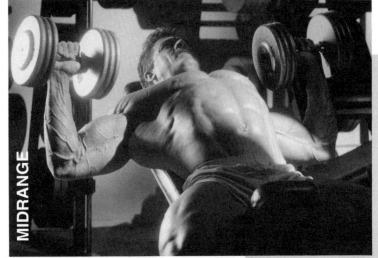
MIDRANGE

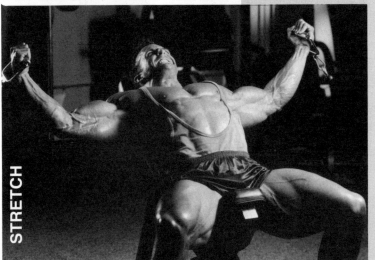
STRETCH

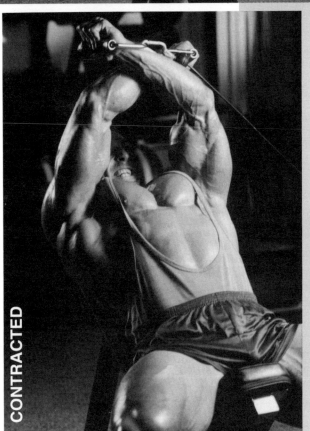
CONTRACTED

## The POF Pec Routine

### Upper chest

*Midrange:*
Incline barbell presses,
　incline dumbbell presses or
　　Smith machine incline presses　　2 x 8-12
(*Include little or no pause at the top or bottom.*)

*Stretch & Contracted:*
Incline cable flyes*　　1-2 x 8-12
(*Pause at the top for two to three seconds for maximum contraction, and at the bottom, or point of stretch, use a quick twitch to enhance the contraction.*)

*For maximum upper-pec contraction make sure that your arms cross at about midforearm. Also, as a substitute for the incline cable flye, a stretch-and-contracted movement, you can do two exercises, one for each position; for example, incline dumbbell flyes for the stretch position and high pec deck flyes or low-cable crossovers—pulling the cables up and crossing your forearms at eye level—for the contracted position. If you choose this route, your upper-chest routine will be as follows:

### Upper chest

*Midrange:*
Incline barbell presses,
　incline dumbbell presses or
　　Smith machine incline presses　　2 x 8-12
(Include little or no pause at the top or bottom.)

*Stretch:* Incline dumbbell flyes*　　1-2 x 8-12
(*At the bottom, or point of stretch, use a quick twitch to involve more muscle fibers.*)

*Contracted:*
High pec deck flyes or
　low-cable crossovers*　　1-2 x 8-12
(*Hold for a two count in the contracted position of each rep.*)

*Note that you don't reach the full contraction on incline dumbbell flyes because there's no resistance in the finish position, and with high pec deck flyes and low-cable crossovers you don't reach the fully stretched position, only the fully contracted position.

### Lower chest

*Midrange:*
Bench presses,
   dumbbell bench presses or
     Smith machine bench presses    2 x 8-12
(*Include little or no pause at the top or bottom.*)

*Stretch & Contracted:*
Decline or
   flat-bench cable flyes or
     cable crossovers\*    1-2 x 8-12
(*Pause at the top for two to three seconds for maximum peak contraction, and at the bottom, or point of stretch, use a quick twitch to involve more muscle fibers.*)

\*For maximum lower-pec contraction make sure your arms cross at about midforearm at the top. As a substitute for decline cable flyes, the stretch-and-contracted movement, you can do two exercises, one for each position; for example, decline dumbbell flyes for the stretch position and pec deck flyes for the contracted position. Your lower-chest routine will look be as follows:

*Midrange:*
Bench presses, dumbbell
   bench presses or Smith machine
   bench presses    2 x 8-12

*Stretch:*
Decline dumbbell flyes\*    1-2 x 8-12

*Contracted:*
Pec deck flyes\*    1-2 x 8-12

\*Note that you don't reach the full contraction on decline dumbbell flyes because there's no resistance in the finish position, and with pec deck flyes you don't reach the fully stretched position, only complete contraction.

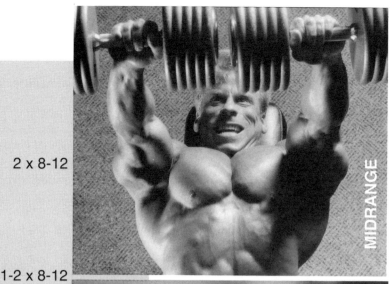

MIDRANGE

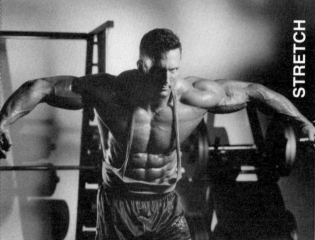

STRETCH

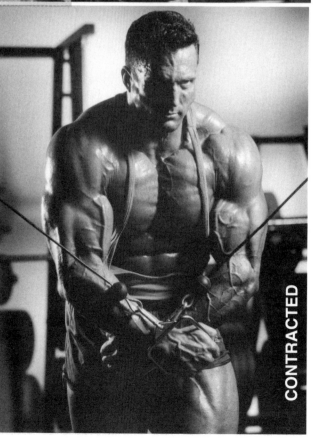

CONTRACTED

With this routine you work your upper chest first to give it priority over the more easily developed (for most trainees) lower-chest. Note also that you completely work your chest with only about eight to 10 sets, a far cry from the 20 to 30 that many bodybuilders use. Remember, if you want maximum growth in minimum time, you have to hit each muscle in an intense, efficient manner and then move on so that you preserve your precious recovery ability for growth.

This strategy should build your chest almost perfectly, and before you know it you'll have the pec power to astonish a poolside crowd with a mere flex and a smile.

## Exercise Descriptions

*Incline barbell presses.* Recline on a 35 degree incline bench with a loaded barbell on the racks behind you. Take a grip that's a little wider than shoulder width on the bar, palms facing forward, and unrack the weight. From this arms-extended position over your chest lower the bar to your clavicles and without a pause drive it back to the top and repeat.

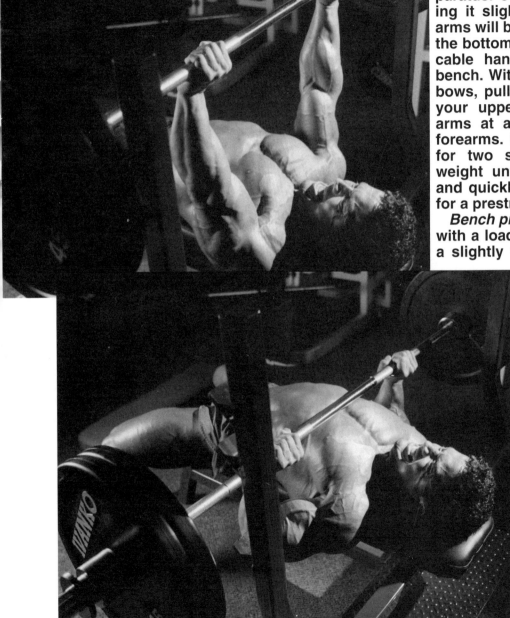

*Incline cable flyes.* Pull a 35 degree incline bench into the crossover apparatus. Center the bench, positioning it slightly forward so that your arms will be pulled down and back at the bottom of each rep. Grab the low cable handles and recline on the bench. With a slight bend in your elbows, pull the handles up and over your upper chest and cross your arms at about the middle of your forearms. Contract your upper pecs for two seconds, then lower the weight until you reach the bottom and quickly reverse your movement for a prestretch. Then repeat.

*Bench presses.* Recline on a bench with a loaded bar on the racks. Take a slightly wider-than-shoulder-width grip on the bar, lift it off of the racks and lower to your middle-chest area. Without pausing, ram the bar back to arm's length and repeat.

*Decline cable flyes.* Pull a decline bench to the center of the crossover apparatus, with the bench positioned slightly forward—again, to where your arms will be pulled down and back at the bottom of each rep. Grab the low handles and recline on the bench. With a slight bend in your elbows, pull the handles until your arms cross at about the middle of your forearms over your abdomen. Contract your lower pecs for two seconds, then lower the weight until you reach the bottom and quickly reverse the movement for a prestretch. Then repeat.

## Critical Chest Q & A

*Q: Incline and decline cable flyes are listed as the stretch-and-contracted-position movements for the upper and lower pecs, respectively. Can I use regular incline and decline dumbbell flyes and get the same results?*

A: Not really, because with dumbbells there's no resistance in the top, or peak-contracted, position, a prerequisite for any contracted-position exercise. Consequently, incline and decline dumbbell flyes are stretch-position movements only. If you use incline and decline dumbbell flyes or flat-bench dumbbell flyes, you should also do a contracted-position movement for each chest area, such as standing low-cable crossovers for your upper chest and pec deck flyes for your lower chest. See the alternate routines. If you train in a home gym and all you have to work with is dumbbells, flex your pecs hard in the top position on flyes and you'll get some peak-contraction benefit.

*Q: Wide-grip dips really seem to stretch my lower pecs. Is this exercise a stretch or midrange movement for the lower pecs?*

A: Although your lower pecs are almost in the stretch position at the bottom of a dip, it's still considered a midrange movement because for most people the deltoids somewhat limit pec stretch at the bottom, when the bend at the elbows is less than 90 degrees. If you're more flexible in your shoulders than most and you can tolerate a slightly wider grip at the lowest point, you can use the dip as a midrange- and stretch-position exercise for your lower pecs. In this case your POF lower-chest routine would be as follows:

*Midrange & Stretch:* Dips     2 x 8-10
*Contracted:* Pec deck flyes     2 x 8-10

Don't forget to use a prestretch at the bottom of each dip.

*Q: If I do my bench presses with dumbbells, won't I hit both the midrange and stretch positions of my lower pecs, since the 'bells allow my hands to go lower than the top of my ribcage?*

A: Once again, the deltoids limit the stretch of the pectorals during this exercise because of the bend in your arms. In order for you to reach the fully stretched position, your hands must be out wide with little or no bend at the elbows, as in a flye. The dumbbell bench press is, therefore, a midrange movement.

*Q: My upper pecs are okay, but my lower pecs really need work. Should I add sets to my lower-pec exercises?*

A: No, don't add sets, or you run the risk of overtraining. Try training your lower chest first in the POF chest routine, and work your upper chest afterward. This will put the priority where you need it, on your lower pecs.

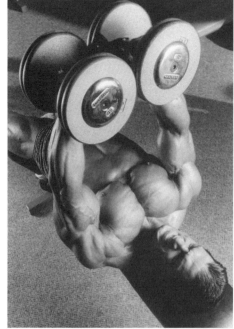

There's no resistance at the top of a dumbbell flye, which makes the cable flye superior when it comes to peak contraction. You can get close to a peak-contraction effect with dumbbells by squeezing at the top of each rep, however.

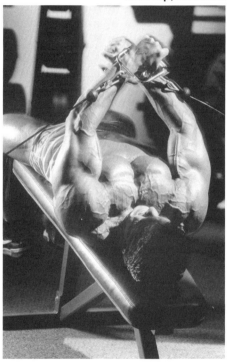

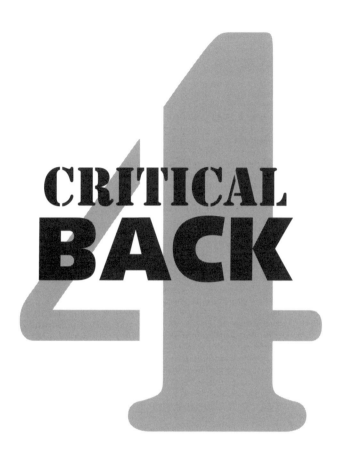

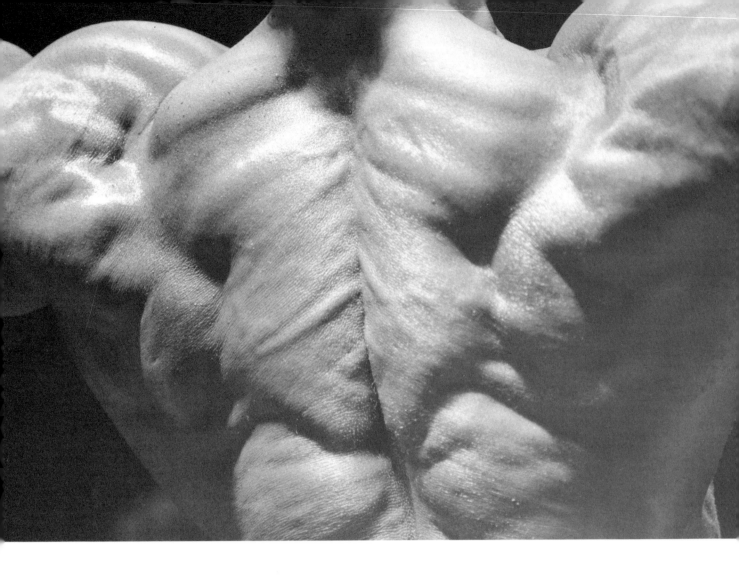
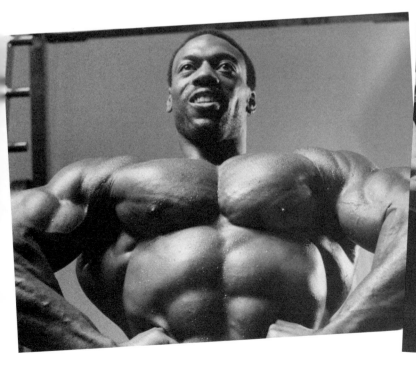
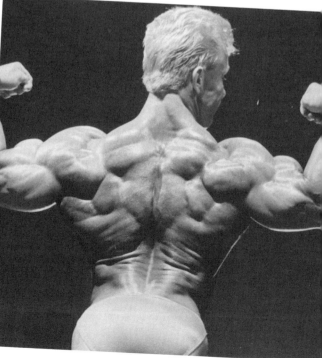

# Building a Back that's Wide, Thick and Majestic

The back is one of the physique's most beautiful yet most rugged areas. When completely developed, this bodypart, with its abundant mounds, deep crevices and sweeping musculature, is a breathtaking work of art—but a work of art with a certain durable quality. Take a look at the photos in this chapter. If you squint your eyes and use a little imagination as you view any one of them, you'll see terrain that would make a mountain climber's mouth water—rugged beauty akin to the mighty Sierras.

The upper back's majesty comes from the numerous smaller muscles that contribute to the functions and appearances of the larger ones. These smaller muscles include the infraspinatus, teres major, teres minor, rhomboideus minor and rhomboideus major, and they're the detailing accessories, so to speak, of the larger trapezius, or midback, and latissimus dorsi, or sweeping outer back.

Because the back has these two very large muscle masses, plus the variety of smaller muscles that fill out the region, most bodybuilders believe that they need to work their backs considerably more than the other bodyparts if they want to attain maximum development. This isn't so, however, because the larger muscles work in conjunction with the smaller ones, and so the smaller muscles don't need any special attention.

## Back Analysis

Even with all of the aforementioned smaller muscles, efficiency-minded bodybuilders will realize that they only have to train the larger masses—the lats and traps. By working these two areas hard and heavy, you hit the smaller muscles just as hard, and they'll become just as developed, especially if you make sure to train the large areas from their three positions of flexion. Using POF enables you to hit every crevice of your back while wasting no effort.

Let's take the two major areas of the upper back, divide each into its three positions of flexion and identify the movements that work each position.

### Latissimus dorsi

*Midrange:* Front chins or front pulldowns—with your upper arms pulling down from overhead and into your sides—work the lats' midrange with help from the biceps and traps. Note that although there's some stretch at the beginning and some contraction with resistance at the end of these movements, you achieve neither position completely, as you'll see from the following descriptions.

*Stretch:* The bottom of a pullover—upper arms overhead with the elbows slightly below the plane of the torso—puts the lats in the total-stretch position. The resistance pulls your arms back, not up, as in a pulldown or chin.

*Contracted:* For you to achieve total peak contraction in your lats, your upper arms must be down, close to and behind your torso, as in the bottom of an undergrip pulldown to the lower chest, a stiff-arm pulldown or a bent-over undergrip row. Scapulae rotation, which you achieve with the aforementioned exercises, is important when you're striving for complete lat contraction.

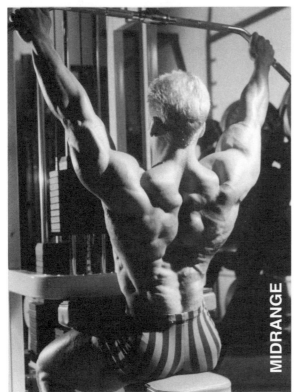

**MIDRANGE**

The pulldown to the front is a midrange movement for the lats.

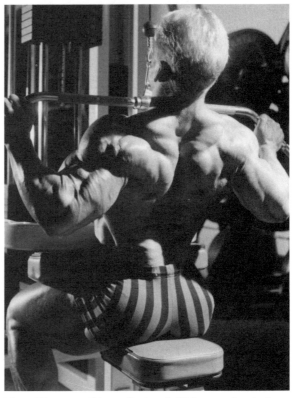

The stiff-arm pulldown (below left) is a contracted-position movement for the lats, and the dumbbell pullover hits the stretch position.

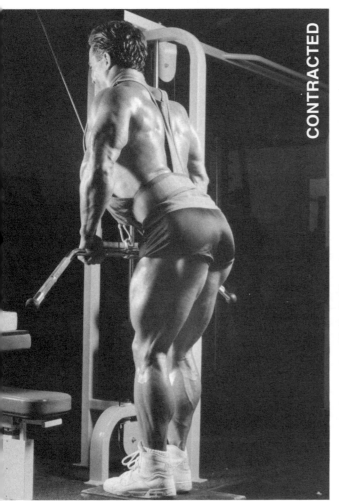

**CONTRACTED**

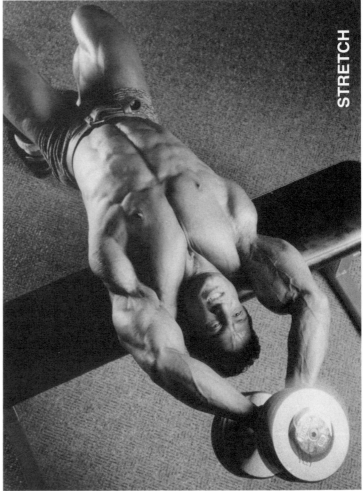

**STRETCH**

### Midback (midtrapezius)

*Midrange:* The behind-the-neck chin or behind-the-neck pulldown with scapulae squeeze works the midrange of the traps with the biceps and lats helping the traps move the resistance. Note that although there is some stretch at the beginning and some contraction at the end of these movements, you reach neither position completely, as you'll see from the following descriptions.

*Stretch:* The bottom of a cable or bent-over row—torso forward and bent at slightly less than 90 degrees to the thighs, arms extended, hands close together—completely stretches the midback. The resistance pulls the arms forward, not up, as in a pulldown.

*Contracted:* The top of a shoulder-width cable row or bent-over row—elbows back behind your torso and angled slightly away from your body and shoulder blades together. With your hands out from your torso and slightly wider than shoulder width apart you provide optimal peak contraction for the midback.

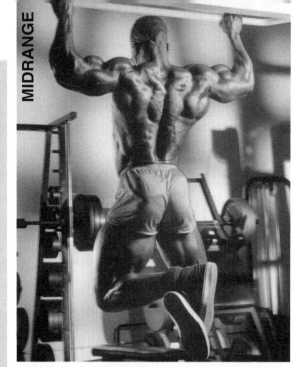

As you can see, hitting the latissimus dorsi's three positions of flexion requires three exercises—front chins, pullovers and stiff-arm pulldowns, for example—while the midback only requires two—behind-the-neck pulldowns and cable rows with the proper handle attachment. The midback needs only two movements because you can work its stretch and contracted positions with one exercise, the cable row, if you use a special separated-handle attachment.

Now, let's construct a productive back attack that will push the bodypart to new levels of width and thickness with as little wasted effort as possible.

### Efficient Back Training

The POF training strategy gives your upper back a thorough workout, but you should follow a couple of rules for best results:

• Work the weaker of the two back areas first. For example, if your midback is fairly well developed but your lats are lagging, work the lats first and the midback second.

• Use a medium-grip—only slightly wider than shoulder width—on all exercises. This will give you a full range of motion.

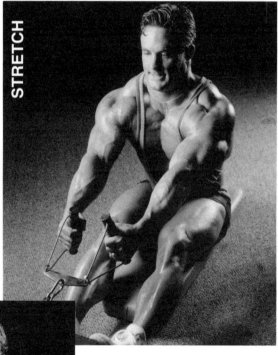

You work the midback's midrange position with behind the neck chins (top). Note how the middle back is engaged in order to pull the body up. You can work the midback's stretch and contracted positions with one movement, the cable row, if you use a separated-handle attachment (above and left) that allows you to start with your hands close together and finish in the contracted position with your hands shoulder width apart.

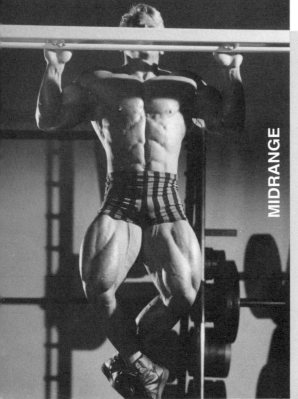

MIDRANGE

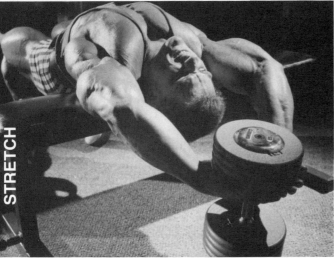

STRETCH

## The POF Back Routine

**Lats**

*Midrange:*
Front pulldowns or chins     2 x 8-12
(*Include little or no pause at the top or bottom.*)

*Stretch:*
Barbell pullovers or dumbbell pullovers*     1-2 x 8-12
(*At the bottom, or point of stretch, use a quick twitch to involve more muscle fibers.*)

*Contracted:*
Undergrip pulldowns,
undergrip bent-over rows
  or stiff-arm pulldowns*     1-2 x 8-12
(*Pause at the bottom for two to three seconds for maximum contraction.*)

*A pullover machine will work both the stretch- and contracted-lat positions. You can substitute this one exercise for pullovers and undergrip pulldowns with the following routine:

*Midrange:*
Front pulldowns
  or chins     2 x 8-12

*Stretch & Contracted:*
Machine pullovers     2 x 8-12

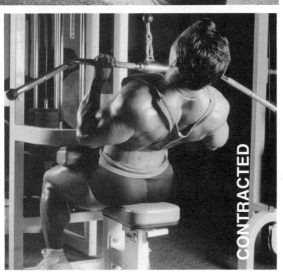

CONTRACTED

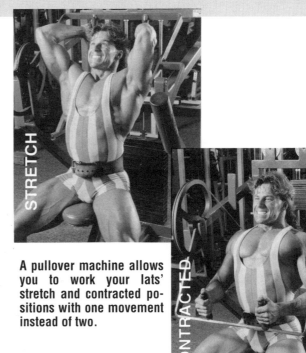

STRETCH / CONTRACTED

A pullover machine allows you to work your lats' stretch and contracted positions with one movement instead of two.

## Midback

*Midrange:*
Behind-the-neck chins     2 x 8-12
(*Include little or no pause at the top or bottom.*)

*Stretch & Contracted:*
Cable rows*
  or two-arm dumbbell rows     2 x 8-12
(*Pause at the top for two or three seconds, and use a quick twitch at the bottom for a more powerful midback contraction.*)

*If you look at the above position descriptions for the midback, you'll see that you should start with your hands close together for complete stretch and end with them slightly wider than shoulder width apart for complete contraction. This is impossible to do when using a bar because your hands are locked in one position. You can achieve it on bent-over rows, however, if you use dumbbells—start with the weights close together, palms facing each other, and end with them wider than your shoulders, palms facing back—or with cable rows if you use a special separated, parallel-handle attachment. In this case start with your hands together for stretch and end with them apart for complete contraction. Note also that although the usual V-handle attachment for cable rows provides a complete stretch, it hinders complete contraction by inhibiting the scapulae squeeze in the finish position.

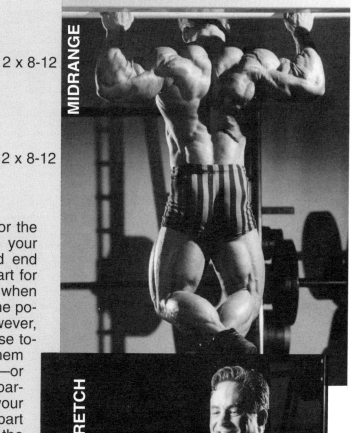

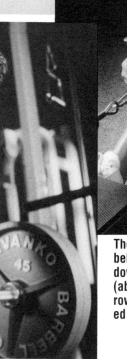

The midback's midrange movement is behind-the-neck chins (top) or pulldowns, while V-handle cable rows (above) and shoulder-width bent-over rows (left) work the stretch and contracted positions, respectively.

STRETCH

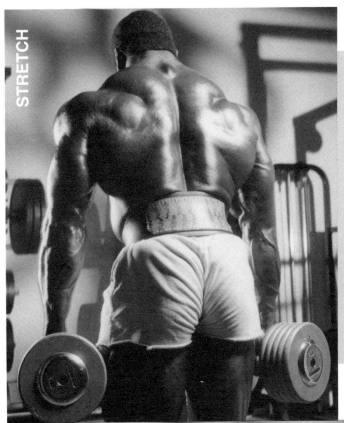

CONTRACTED

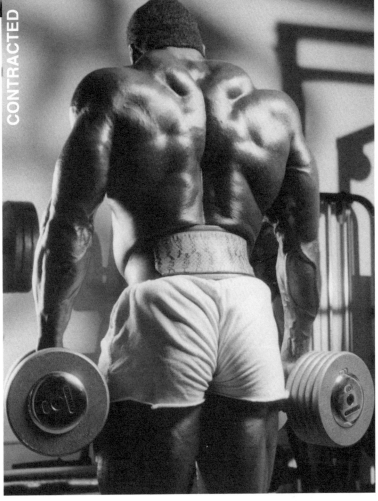

### Upper Traps

*Stretch & Contracted:*
Barbell or dumbbell shrugs
  with a forward lean*    2 x 8-10
(*Pause for two to three seconds at the top, and use a quick twitch at the bottom for a more powerful trap contraction.*)

*You train your upper traps, which tend to work somewhat independently of the middle traps, at the end of your back routine because you've already hit their midrange position with behind-the-neck pulldowns. Note, however, that you should only do shrugs if you need upper-trap work, which refers to the area from your shoulders to your neck. Most bodybuilders get plenty of indirect stimulation in that area from other delt and back exercises.)

Keep in mind that this is an intermediate-advanced routine. At the top end you do 12 sets, which is quite a bit of work, so unless you're advanced, skip the shrugs and stick to the lower set numbers for eight total sets.

There's no denying that POF covers all the angles and provides a mind-blowing, back-growing pump. If you're interested in complete back development achieved with efficiency in the gym, give this routine a try. There's one drawback though: You may have mountain climbers wanting to have a go at that rugged terrain you call your upper back.

Shrugs with a forward lean enable you to work both the stretch and contracted positions of your upper traps.

## Exercises Descriptions

*Front pulldowns.* Take a grip on the pulldown bar with your hands slightly wider than your shoulders. Anchor your legs under the supports, get comfortable and pull the bar down to your clavicles. Keep a relatively upright position—no leaning back. A slight lower-back arch is acceptable, but don't turn it into a rowing movement.

*Barbell pullovers.* Recline on a flat bench with your head hanging off of one end and a loaded EZ-curl bar on the floor behind you. Grab the bar with a shoulder-width grip and your palms facing up. With your arms bent, pull the bar up over your head to your chest, keeping it about two inches from your face. Touch your upper chest with it, return to the starting position along the same arc, and reverse the movement at the bottom with a prestretch twitch. Repeat.

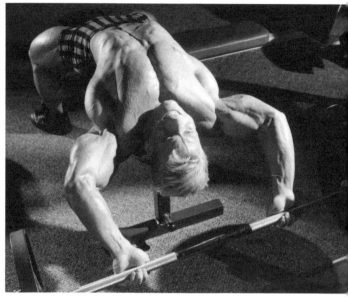

*Undergrip pulldowns.* Grab the pulldown bar with a shoulder-width grip and your palms facing back toward you. Secure your thighs under the supports and pull the bar down to your lower chest as you lean back. As much as a 45 degree lean is acceptable. You also want to arch your lower back on this exercise to enhance scapulae rotation. Because of the undergrip your arms remain close to your torso, and there's no danger of this turning into a rowing exercise as there is with regular pulldowns to the front. Your elbows should be back behind your torso at the end of the range of motion so the lats are fully contracted.

*Behind-the-neck pulldowns.* Take a slightly wider-than-shoulder-width grip on the pulldown bar with your palms facing forward. Pull the bar down while you squeeze your shoulder blades together. Don't lean too far forward. When it touches the base of your neck, extend your arms slowly and repeat.

*Cable rows.* For proper stretch and contraction on this exercise it's best to use two separate handles that will allow your hands to spread apart in the top position so you can completely contract your midback. To perform the exercise, sit on the cable row platform, grab the separate handles and lean forward slightly with your hands together to feel a stretch in your midback. Pull the handles toward your abdomen, and spread your hands as you reach your torso, keeping your arms slightly up and away from your sides while simultaneously sitting upright. Don't let your torso go beyond a 90 degree angle to the bench. Hold this position at your abdomen and squeeze your shoulder blades together for two seconds, then release slowly as you lean forward. As you reach the stretch position, let your hands come together and then reverse the movement with a quick twitch and begin another rep. Repeat. Note that despite the common gym practice, you shouldn't squeeze your arms into the sides of your body in the contracted position, because it works too much lat. Keep your arms slightly up and away from your sides to fully contract your midback muscles.

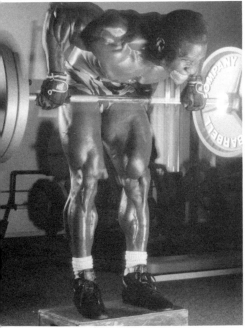

The bent-over row is a contracted-position movement for the midback.

When you do cable rows with your arms in close to your torso, you target your lats, not your midback, because it puts your lats in the contracted position.

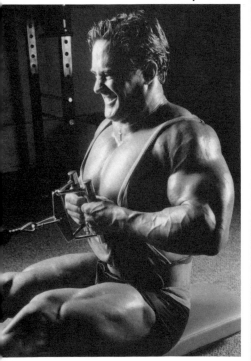

## Critical Back Q & A

*Q: I really like bent-over barbell rows. How can I incorporate them into the POF strategy?*

*A:* Use them as a contracted-position movement and include a close-grip rowing exercise as your stretch-position movement. Here's an example:

| | |
|---|---|
| *Midrange:* Behind-the-neck pulldowns | 2 x 8-10 |
| *Stretch:* Close-grip cable rows (separated handles) | 2 x 8-10 |
| *Contracted:* Bent-over barbell rows | 1-2 x 8-10 |

Be sure to use a grip that's slightly wider than shoulder width, take a two-second pause at the top for maximum midback contraction and keep your arms out away from your torso for the greatest possible scapulae squeeze.

*Q: If I do my cable or bent-over rows with my arms in close to my body, am I working more lat or midback?*

*A:* When you pull your arms in close to your torso, you change the emphasis of this exercise from your midback to your lats. Notice that at the end of these movements you're in the lats' contracted position. Feel free to use the arms-in version of cable or bent-over rows as a contracted-position lat movement every so often; however, you might want to use an undergrip to help keep your arms in the proper position and for more advantageous leverage. Here's a sample lat routine:

| | |
|---|---|
| *Midrange:* Pulldowns | 2 x 8-10 |
| *Stretch:* Pullovers | 2 x 8-10 |
| *Contracted:* Undergrip cable rows | 1-2 x 8-10 |

*Q: I have an injured shoulder and can't do behind-the-neck pulldowns, the midrange exercise for the middle back. Is there a substitute?*

*A:* Yes and no. The only real substitute for behind-the-neck pulldowns in this instance is cable crossover pulldowns. You grab the crossover handles, kneel on the floor with your torso upright and pull the handles down toward your shoulders. Squeeze your shoulder blades together at the bottom, release slowly and repeat. The reason this isn't quite as good a midrange middle-back movement is that it really works only the lower midrange and tends to bring in the lats more than behind-the-neck pulldowns do. It will suffice, however, and keep you from further shoulder damage. If you still feel stress in that area, skip the midrange movement altogether until you're completely healed and concentrate on the stretch and contracted positions. For more on your shoulder problems and how to rehabilitate them, get a copy of Health For Life's *The 7-Minute Rotator Cuff Solution.*

*Q: My gym has a Nautilus behind-the-neck torso machine, the one on which the pads are against your triceps and you pull your arms from overhead down to your sides in an arc.*

This exercise simulates a pulldown but without bringing the arms into play. Is it a midrange-, stretch- or contracted-position movement for the lats?

A: Some people would classify the behind-the-neck torso movement as either a stretch- or contracted-position exercise at first glance, but before you jump to this conclusion, consider two things: 1) The finish position is not the completely contracted position for the lats—your arms are down, but they're not back behind the torso, as in the finish position of an undergrip pulldown, so there's no scapulae rotation; and 2) in the start position the resistance pushes your arms together overhead, not back behind the plane of your torso, where they should be in the stretch position. The behind-the-neck torso machine movement is, therefore, a midrange lat exercise, similar to the front pulldown, although the synergy is minimized because your biceps are taken out of the movement.

Q: Can I do wide-grip chins or pulldowns for my midrange lat movement instead of using a shoulder-width grip?

A: Although your range of motion will be more limited, for variety's sake go ahead and use a wider grip. Don't go too wide, however, or you could damage your shoulder.

Q: I tend to feel bent-over laterals in my middle back rather than my rear delts. Is this exercise a back movement?

A: Yes, and it's a good one at that. If you keep your arms bent and squeeze your scapulae together at the top, you have a midback contracted-position exercise. At the top you'll look as if you're doing a wide-grip bent-over row. In other words, the bends in your elbows should be very severe so you can effectively squeeze your scapulae together. If you do this exercise with little or no bend in your elbows, you work primarily your rear-delt heads.

Don't think, however, that because you start the movement with your hands close together, it's also a stretch-position movement. Unfortunately, you have to pull the weight toward you to work the midback's stretch position, as in cable rows, not out in an arc. If you want to incorporate bent-arm bent-over laterals into your POF back strategy, you can alter the previous routine, as follows:

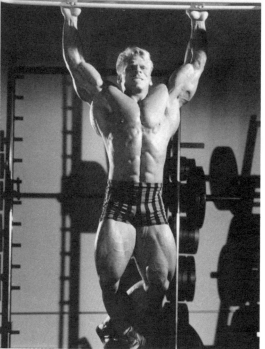

A wider grip on chins and pulldowns limits your range of motion, but periodic grip changes are, nevertheless, good for variety.

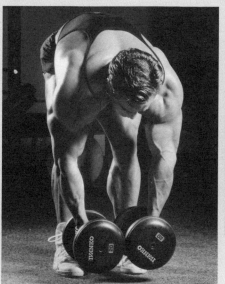

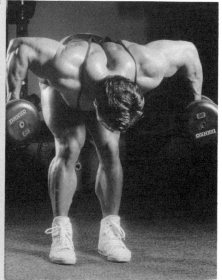

Bent-arm bent-over laterals enable you to squeeze your midback for maximum peak contraction.

| | |
|---|---|
| *Midrange:* Behind-the-neck pulldowns | 2 x 8-10 |
| *Stretch:* Close parallel-grip cable rows (V-handle) | 2 x 8-10 |
| *Contracted:* Bent-arm bent-over lateral raises | 1 x 8-10 |

*Q: Wouldn't bent-over cable laterals, on which the arms cross, put the midback in more of a stretch position than bent-over dumbbell rows or cable rows, on which the hands are still somewhat apart?*

*A:* Because the angle of pull is to the sides on bent-over cable laterals, the rear delts are the prime movers, not the midback. At the top the resistance is still pulling to the sides, which also puts the trapezius at a disadvantage. Therefore, you should avoid cable laterals unless you're looking for a rear-delt exercise and concentrate on cable rows with separate handles or bent-over two-arm dumbbell rows, which will effectively work both the stretch and contracted positions. Note that in the peak-contracted positions of these exercises, the resistance is straight down, as it should be for a proper midback contraction.

*Q: I train at home and don't have access to a pulldown machine. Is there another exercise I can use other than stiff-arm pulldowns to isolate my lats and work their contracted position?*

*A:* Yes, you can use bent-over scapulae rotations. Take a dumbbell in each hand and bend over at the waist, with your torso parallel to the floor and your arms extended as if you were going to do bent-over laterals. Pull the dumbbells back toward you and up into what resembles the finish position of a kickback but with your arms slightly bent. This provides scapulae rotation and puts you in the lats' contracted position. Note that your upper arms must be past your torso in the contracted position and should remain slightly bent to avoid too much triceps involvement.

*Q: Are one-arm bent-over dumbbell rows a stretch- and contracted-position movement for the midback?*

*A:* No, but they're a very good stretch-position exercise. The reason they don't qualify as a contracted-position movement is because of torso rotation. At the top of the movement, when you're close to peak contraction, your torso tends to roll away from the dumbbell. This inhibits midback contraction and puts one-arm bent-over dumbbell rows in the midback-stretch-position category. If you like one-arm dumbbell rows, here's how you can incorporate them into your POF midback strategy:

| | |
|---|---|
| *Midrange:* Behind-the-neck pulldowns | 2 x 8-10 |
| *Stretch:* One-arm bent-over rows | 2 x 8-10 |
| *Contracted:* Bent-arm bent-over laterals | 1 x 8-10 |

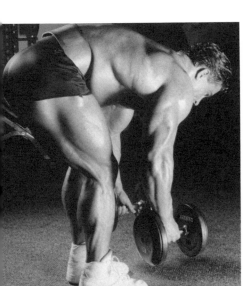

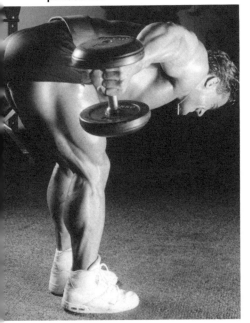

You can use bent-over scapulae rotations to work your lats' contracted position if you don't have access to a machine for stiff-arm pulldowns.

# 5 CRITICAL DELTS

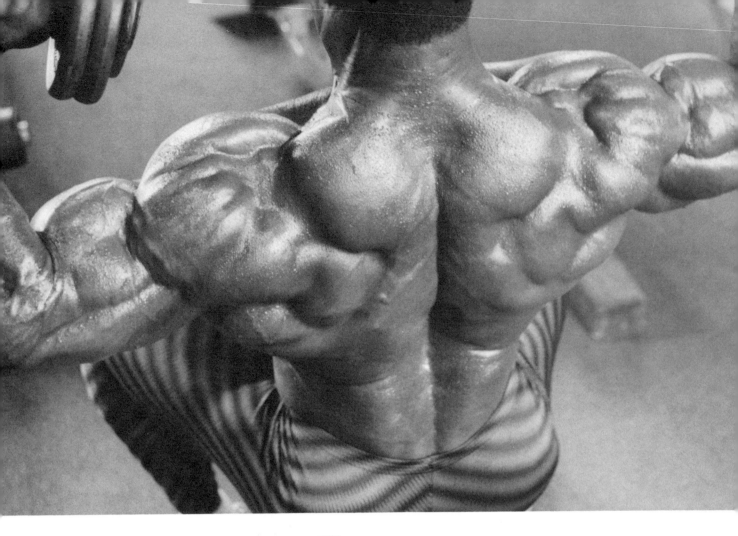
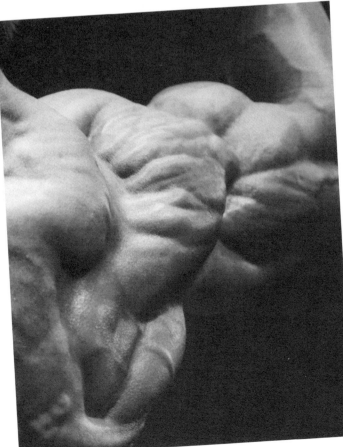
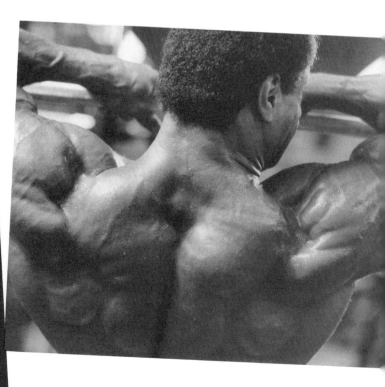

# A Boulder Approach

Cannonballs. Boulders. The twin planets. No matter what you call your shoulders, one thing is certain: With a power-packed pair of delts you'll feel as though you can command the universe.

There's something about wide, round shoulders that gives bodybuilders a mighty and powerful demeanor. Can you imagine Shawn Ray or Gary Strydom strutting around without their devastating deltoid development? It's not a pretty picture. When bodybuilders are lacking in the delt department, they look slump shouldered, narrow and just plain destitute.

Fortunately, a little muscle goes a long way when it comes to delts. All it takes is a small amount of added mass on each lateral, or side, head to boost a bodybuilder's torso from mediocre to Herculean.

If that's all it takes, why are there so many bodybuilders with shriveled shrimp shoulders instead of cannonballs crowning their clavicles? It could be an epidemic of bad genetics, but more often than not we can pin the problem on overtraining.

## Overtraining: the Delt Destroyer

The lateral-deltoid head is a rather small muscle—even smaller than the biceps. It's in such an important position when it comes to bodybuilding, however, that it's often bombarded with excessive work in a desperate attempt to create more width and roundness. In the case of a small muscle like the lateral-delt head, the additional work usually means stagnation or even a loss of mass; the muscle simply can't recover and grow, so it stays in a constant state of catch-up and often breaks down instead of building up.

To keep from driving yourself into this overtrained state, you must make your delt work as efficient and precise as possible—efficient in that it should utilize the least amount of work necessary to stimulate maximum growth and precise in that it should primarily stress the important lateral heads. If you have a knowledge of anatomy, however, you may be wondering about the other two delt heads.

While it's true that the deltoid is made up of three heads—anterior, or front; lateral; and posterior, or rear—it's also true that the front and rear heads get so much work from other exercises that they rarely need direct stimulation. For example, any type of press, flye or curl works the front heads to a degree, while pulldowns, rows and chins work the rear heads. Also, remember that no muscle is an island, especially when it's in as close proximity to other muscles as the three delt heads are. This being the case, any lateral-head exercise—such as lateral raises—indirectly affects the other two heads.

As for any indirect stimulation of the lateral head from other exercises, it doesn't get nearly as much and therefore must be blasted from all angles with sharpshooter precision if you want dramatic density and fullness.

## Precision Training With POF

Most bodybuilders' delt training has about as much accuracy as a sawed-off shotgun on a bird-hunting expedition; more often than not it misses the mark completely, but when it does nail the small target, it disintegrates the meat beyond recognition. In order to hit all the angles, the average bodybuilder attempts to use every shoulder exercise in the book, which causes an overtrained, overdrained state that limits, rather than promotes, gains.

Let's take the lateral deltoid and dissect its three positions to determine exercises that work each.

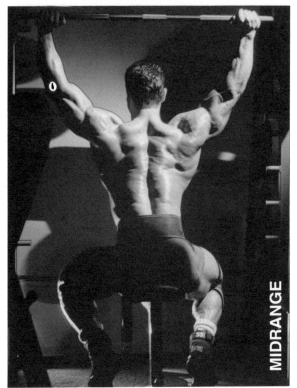

Midrange delt exercises include any of the overhead pressing movements.

*Midrange:* Overhead pressing movements focus on the midrange position—you don't achieve full stretch or full contraction. The triceps and traps help the deltoids move the resistance.

*Stretch:* The bottom of a one-arm incline lateral raise or one-arm cable lateral—arm across the front of the torso—puts the lateral head in the stretch position.

*Contracted:* The top position of an upright row or lateral raise—upper arm out to the side and angled slightly upward—completely contracts the lateral head.

Once you understand these three positions, precise, efficient delt training is simply a matter of devising a routine that forces your shoulders into the growth zone at every workout without disrupting your recovery ability. If you're an intermediate-to-advanced bodybuilder, you'll have the recovery ability to handle more sets than a beginner can, but you still can't overdo it without suffering the overtraining consequences. Remember, the lateral head is a small muscle and doesn't require all that much work to get it growing. Here's an excellent delt routine that hits the POF highlights:

You work the contracted position of your delts with lateral raises and the stretch position with incline lateral raises. Note that on the incline laterals your arm comes across your torso so that your lateral-delt head is stretched at the bottom.

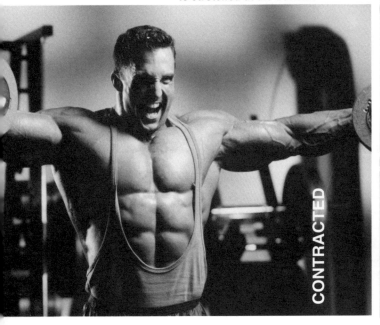

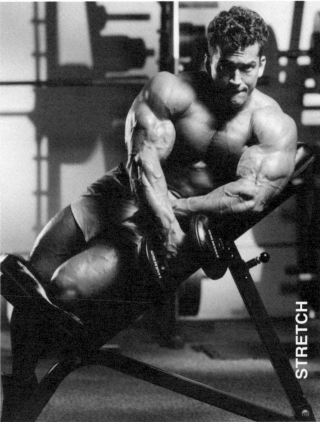

66 Critical Mass

## POF Delt Routine

*Midrange:*
Behind-the-neck presses,
　dumbbell presses, military presses
　　or Arnold presses　　　　　　　2 x 8-12
(*Include little or no pause at the top or bottom.*)

*Stretch:*
Incline one-arm lateral raises
　or one-arm cable lateral raises　　2 x 8-12
(*At the bottom, or point of stretch, use a quick twitch for a more intense delt contraction.*)

*Contracted:*
Wide-grip upright rows,
　lateral raises or one-arm leaning
　　lateral raises　　　　　　　　1-2 x 8-12
(*Pause at the top of each rep for two seconds for maximum contraction.*)

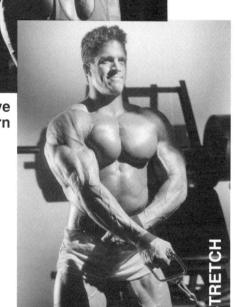

At the high end you do six sets, which is probably more than enough work for the lateral-delt head if you work at least to positive failure on each.

If you're interested in a pair of devastating delts that have dynamite density, give the POF approach a try. It will turn your shoulders into boulders in no time.

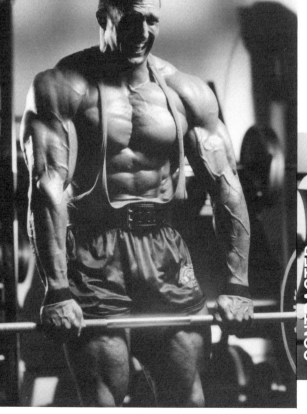

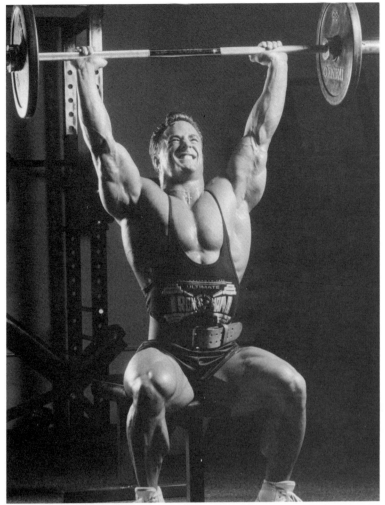

## Exercises Descriptions

*Behind-the-neck presses.* Take a loaded barbell off a rack and place it across your shoulders as if you were going to do squats. Sit on a bench, plant your feet on the floor and press the barbell overhead. Lower the bar to the back of your neck below ear level and repeat.

*Incline one-arm lateral raises.* Sit sideways on an incline bench, lean one shoulder against the bench and work your other shoulder with a one-arm lateral raise, lifting the dumbbell across your torso and up. The incline lets the lateral delt get a full stretch in the bottom position. Keep the dumbbell tipped slightly forward at all times, holding your pinkie a little higher than your thumb. Also, don't forget that this is a stretch-position exercise, which means you shouldn't pause at the bottom but instead quickly reverse the movement in order to take advantage of the prestretch phenomenon and involve as many muscle fibers as possible.

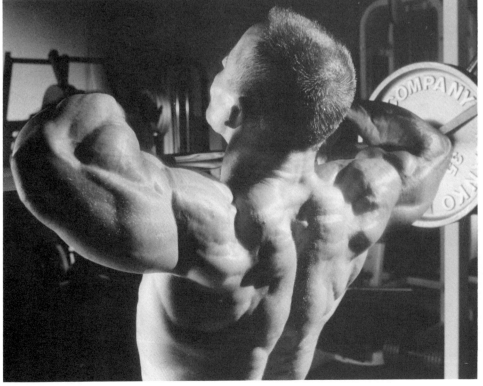

*Wide-grip upright rows.* Use a slightly wider-than-shoulder-width grip. While standing upright with the barbell hanging at arm's length, pull it up to your chest, keeping it close to your body. Stop at midchest level for two seconds, then lower slowly and repeat. If this exercise hurts your wrists or shoulders, use dumbbells for less joint restriction.

## Critical Delts Q & A

*Q: I like to do a version of lateral raises with the low cables. It's like performing one-arm cable laterals only with both arms at once. Does this movement work the delts' stretch and contracted positions?*

*A:* At first glance you'd think so, but because of the angle of pull, it's only a stretch-position movement. When you reach the top, you're pulling out more instead of up. Consequently, you aren't effectively working the contracted position during this exercise—the traps are doing a lot of the work. The resistance should pull straight down at the top of the range of motion, as in a dumbbell lateral raise, to make the exercise a true contracted-position movement for the lateral-deltoid heads.

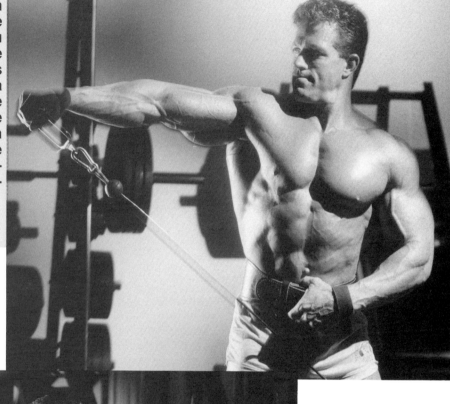

Note how on cable laterals (right) the trainee tends to shrug his shoulder because the angle of pull is off to the side. This diffuses the peak-contraction effect somewhat and places stress on the traps. With regular laterals (below) the resistance pulls straight down, which forces the delts to maintain most of the stress in the contracted position.

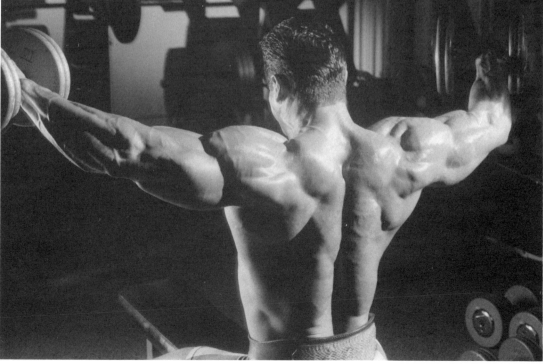

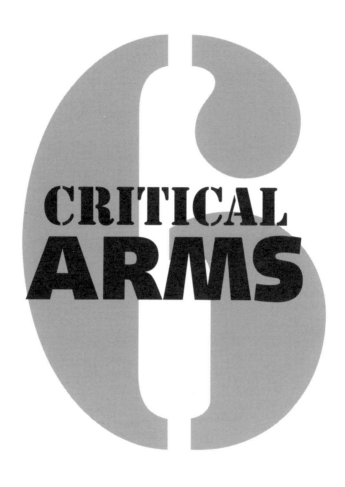

# CRITICAL ARMS

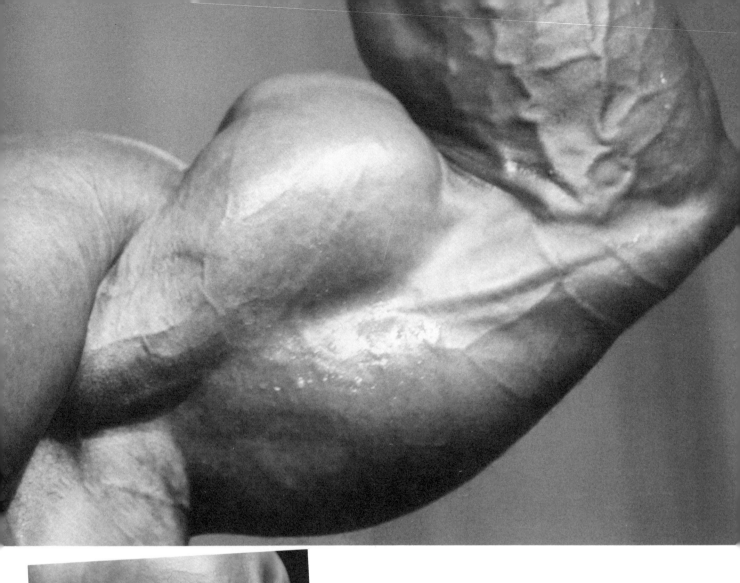
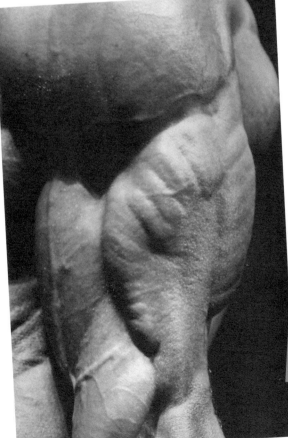
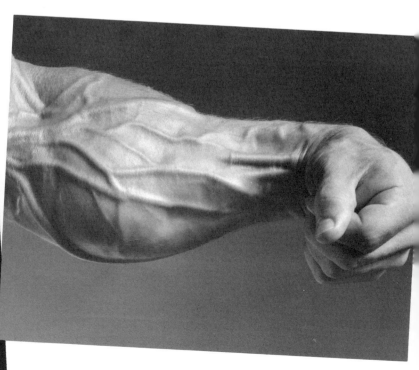

# Shoulder-to-Wrist Growth Blitz

Arms are a bodybuilder's credentials. A set of gargantuan guns gives notice that the owner pumps some serious iron and is proud of it. The triceps' illustrious sweep, the biceps' jutting magnificence and the forearms' vascular fullness cause men, women and even beasts to do a double take when they see this development hanging precariously out of a short-sleeved shirt.

Even for the more worldly average Joe, seeing Mike Matarazzo, Lee Haney or even Arnold in slacks and a polo shirt can be an inspiring—if not intimidating—experience. While the tailored fabric hides the musculature of the torso, thighs and calves, giving the bodybuilder an almost normal appearance, when eyes meet arms, the reaction turns to shock. Two ominous appendages cascade out of the shirtsleeves, each resembling a side of beef that could easily feed a family of 15. Once the shock subsides, the envy eventually sets in. To have admirable arm development is a dream of almost every man—and even a number of women—on the planet.

In 1960, for example, Tony Curtis was one of the stars of "Spartacus," along with actor extraordinaire Laurence Olivier. After the two had filmed a few shirtless scenes, Olivier asked Curtis point blank how he got such extraordinary arms. It seems that Olivier had always wanted a set like Curtis' for himself. Now, Curtis' arms were nowhere near the size of today's physique champs, but back in the B.A. (Before Arnold) era they were considered above average. Well-developed arms have always been, and will always be, an admired possession.

## The Arms Race

Because great guns are universally admired, getting them is usually the neophyte bodybuilder's first goal. All other bodyparts become secondary. In the beginning arms get an abundance of blow-torching, while other bodyparts are put on the back burner, so to speak. This can be a somewhat dangerous circumstance to the aspiring bodybuilder because the overwork can bring slow, stunted growth. Sure, the arms will grow—to a point—but hypertrophy eventually stops and can even begin to regress after too many marathon efforts.

Remember that the forearms, biceps and triceps get more secondary work than any other muscle group. Triceps get it from pressing, biceps get it from pulling—as in rows and chins—and forearms get it from hanging and gripping. When you add set after set of direct arm work to your routine, you eventually run into diminishing returns. The key to awesome arms is simple. Train them intensely, efficiently and not too frequently.

## Arm Yourself With POF

Logic will tell you that there's no need to do an endless number of arm movements in order to "hit all the angles." It's simply a waste of time and precious energy. It's much more logical to figure out how each muscle or muscle group works, blitz each angle with one or two high-intensity sets and then move on to the next bodypart. If you do this on a consistent basis, total development will be yours in much less time.

As usual, we'll start with a bodypart analysis. Here are the major arm muscles and how their specific positions of flexion break down:

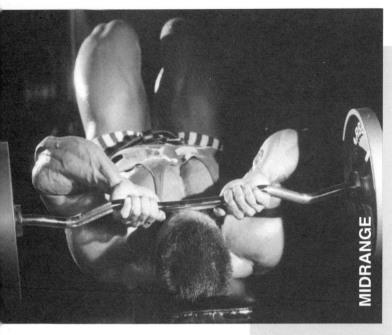
*MIDRANGE*

## Triceps

*Midrange:* You achieve this position when your arm is straight out in front of you, perpendicular to your torso, as in lying triceps extensions. When you do that exercise correctly, with some upper-arm movement, your lats become synergists, assisting your triceps in moving the resistance.

*Stretch:* Maximum triceps stretch occurs when your upper arm is next to the side of your head and your lower arm is bent back behind it, with your knuckles almost touching your shoulder, as in the bottom of a standing triceps extension.

*Contracted:* You reach total triceps contraction when your arm is down next to your side and slightly back behind your body with your elbow locked—with the muscle fully flexed. Triceps kickbacks or one-arm pushdowns work this position.

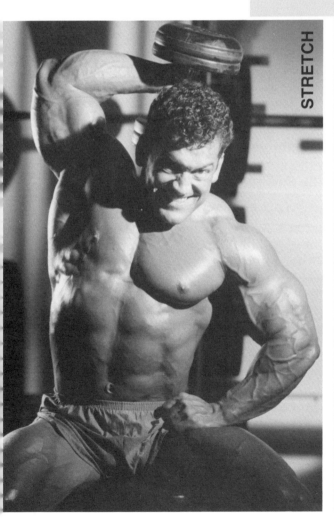
*STRETCH*

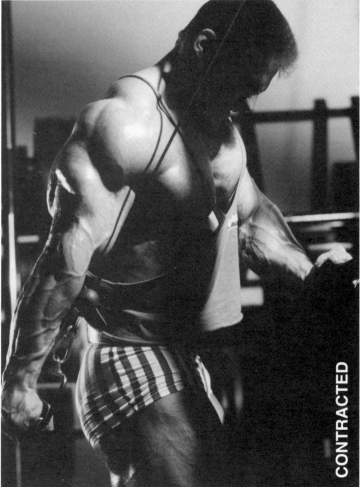
*CONTRACTED*

## Biceps

*Midrange:* You hit this position when your upper arm is slightly in front of your torso, as in standing barbell curls or preacher curls. The front delt helps the biceps in both of these exercises, more so in standing barbell curls, as your arms travel slightly forward while you curl the bar up.

*Stretch:* You get complete biceps stretch when your upper arm is straight down and back behind the plane of your torso, as in the bottom of a low-incline dumbbell curl.

*Contracted:* Your biceps is fully contracted when your upper arm is next to your head, your forearm flush against your upper arm, with your palm down and your little finger twisting outward. This position is hard to simulate with any conventional barbell exercise, although you could conceivably do a one-arm behind-the-head cable curl. Since that would be somewhat awkward to perform, use nonsupport concentration curls to get you as close as possible to the contracted position.

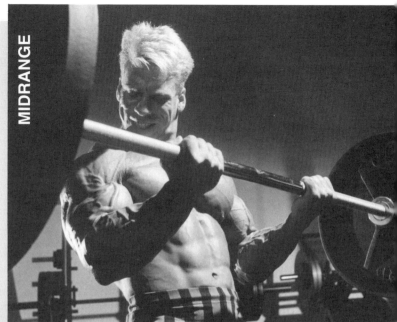

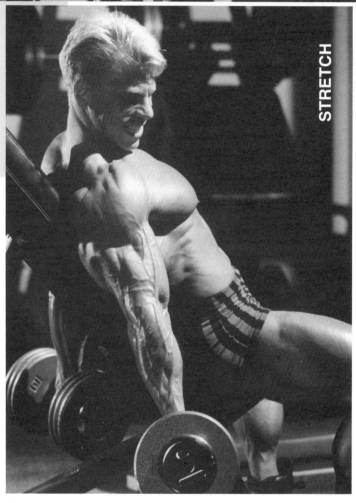

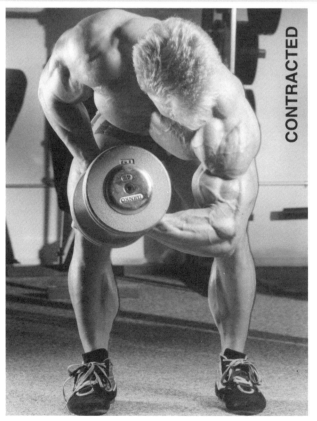

Nonsupport concentration curls (left) don't quite allow you to reach the biceps' completely contracted position, but they'll get you very close.

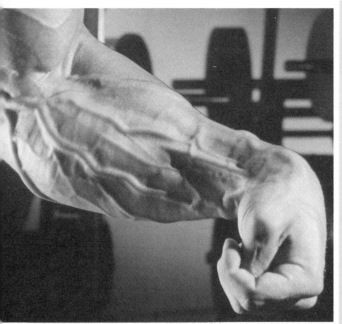

The forearm flexors are the beefy underside of the lower arm (above), while the forearm extensors run along the top of the lower arm (below).

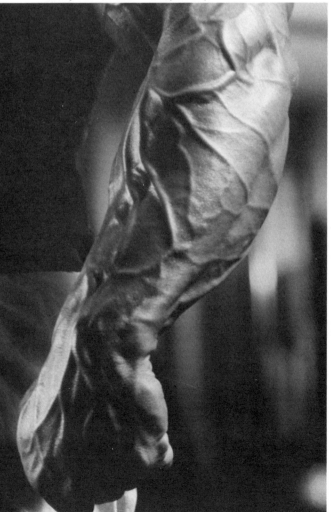

**Forearms (flexors: underside)**

*Midrange:* This position gets worked with all the gripping you do and the movement that occurs when you perform other exercises, specifically any type of curl, so there's no need to target it directly in your forearm program.

*Stretch:* You get complete forearm flexor stretch in the bottom position of a palms-up wrist curl when you're sitting on a bench that's angled slightly upward, your forearms are resting on the bench, and the bend in your elbow is greater than 90 degrees.

*Contracted:* You can completely contract your forearm flexors in the top position of a palms-up wrist curl when you're sitting on a bench that's angled slightly downward and the bend in your elbow is less than 90 degrees.

**Forearms (extensors: top of forearm)**

*Midrange:* You work this position with reverse curls. The biceps help pull the forearm extensors through the midrange position.

*Stretch:* You completely stretch your forearm extensors in the bottom position of a reverse wrist curl when you're sitting on a bench that's angled slightly upward, your forearms are resting on the bench, and the bend in your elbow is greater than 90 degrees.

*Contracted:* You achieve complete contraction in your forearm extensors in the top position of a reverse wrist curl when you're sitting on a bench that's angled slightly downward, your forearms are resting on the bench, and the bend in your elbow is less than 90 degrees to allow for better contraction.

The protocol for precise arm training is simple. Pick one exercise for each position, train it intensely and watch your arms blossom rapidly to side-of-beef proportions. A complete shoulder-to-wrist POF arm blitz looks like this:

## POF Arm Routine

**Triceps**

*Midrange:*
Lying triceps extensions
  or close-grip bench presses        2 x 8-12
(*Include little or no pause at the top or bottom.*)

*Stretch:*
Overhead extensions or cable
  pushouts (from a lunging position)  2 x 8-12
(*At the bottom, or point of stretch, use a quick twitch for a more intense triceps contraction.*)

*Contracted:*
Dumbbell kickbacks, one-arm cable kickbacks
  or one-arm triceps pushdowns
    (upper arm behind torso)          1 x 8-12
(*Pause at the top of each rep for two seconds for maximum contraction.*)

**Biceps**

*Midrange:*
Barbell curls, seated dumbbell
  curls or preacher curls             2 x 8-12
(*Include little or no pause at the top or bottom.*)

*Stretch:*
Incline dumbbell curls or one-arm
  cable curls (upper arm behind torso)  2 x 8-12
(*At the bottom, or point of stretch, use a quick twitch for a more intense biceps contraction.*)

*Contracted:*
One-arm concentration curls,
  barbell concentration curls or spider curls  1 x 8-12
(*Pause at the top of each rep for two seconds.*)

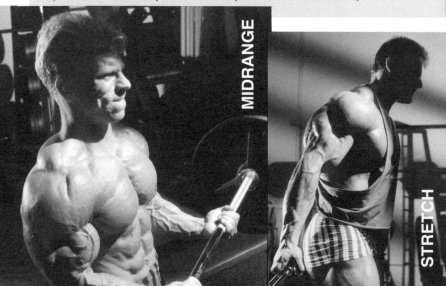
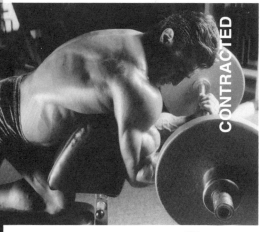

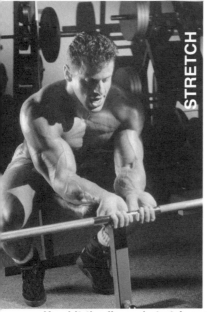
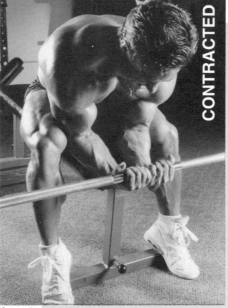

### Forearm flexors

*Midrange:*
Worked during biceps curls.

*Stretch:*
Incline wrist curls  1 x 8-12
(*At the bottom, or point of stretch, instead use a quick twitch for a more intense forearm flexor contraction.*)

*Contracted:* Decline wrist curls  1 x 8-12
(*Pause at the top of each rep for two seconds.*)

### Forearm extensors

*Midrange:*
Reverse curls or hammer curls  1 x 8-12
(*Include little or no pause at the top or bottom.*)

*Stretch:*
Incline reverse wrist curls  1 x 8-12
(*At the bottom, or point of stretch, use a quick twitch for a more intense forearm extensor contraction.*)

*Contracted:*
Decline reverse wrist curls  1 x 8-12
(*Pause at the top of each rep for two seconds.*)

You hit the flexors' stretch position at the bottom of an incline wrist curl when the angle at your elbows is greater than 90 degrees. You reach the contracted position at the top of a decline wrist curl when the angle at your elbows is less than 90 degrees.

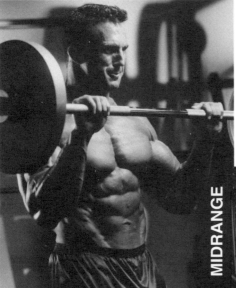
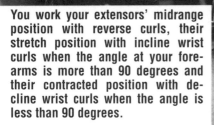

You work your extensors' midrange position with reverse curls, their stretch position with incline wrist curls when the angle at your forearms is more than 90 degrees and their contracted position with decline wrist curls when the angle is less than 90 degrees.

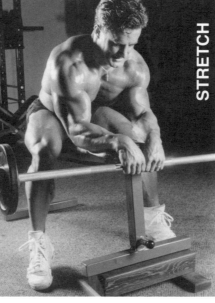
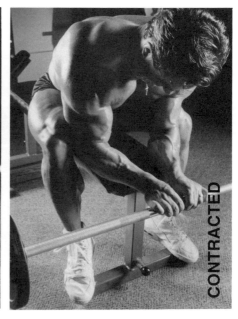

Here are a few pointers to help you get the most out of POF arm training:

• Train triceps before biceps. If you do biceps first, the pumped muscles will act as a forearm buffer and prevent a full range of motion on some triceps movements. For example, if you do overhead triceps extensions with pumped biceps, your range of motion will be somewhat limited in the low, or stretch, position.

• Train forearms last so that you don't fatigue your gripping muscles and inhibit your performance of other exercises.

• Try to maintain a relatively slow pace on every exercise—two seconds up and two seconds down is as fast as you should move. This speed will help you feel the muscle working during each rep and prevent you from using momentum, which could cause injury.

As a side note, in Arnold's heyday his favorite biceps routine was incline dumbbell curls, standing dumbbell curls and nonsupport concentration curls. Whether he realized it or not, he was using POF. The inclines worked his biceps' stretch position, the standing dumbbell curls hit their midrange position, and the nonsupport concentration curls got the contracted position. And Arnold had a pair of the greatest biceps the world has ever seen.

The key to out-of-this-world arms is a regimen of precise, intense workouts. If you want your guns to cause people's jaws to drop, give the POF arm blitz a try.

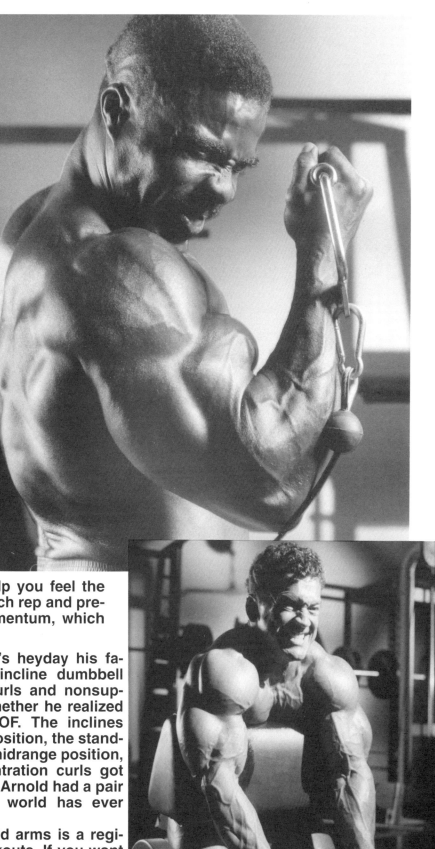

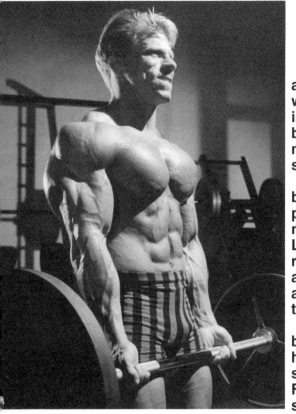

## Exercise Descriptions

*Barbell curls.* Stand upright with a loaded barbell at arm's length. Slowly curl the bar up to your shoulders without swinging your body. Some upper-arm movement is fine, as this brings the front-deltoid heads into play, but you don't want momentum to carry the weight. Remember, this is a midrange exercise, so there should be synergy.

*Incline dumbbell curls.* Recline on a 45-degree-incline bench with a dumbbell in each hand. From a dead-hang position curl the dumbbells up to your shoulder simultaneously with as little upper-arm movement as possible. Lower and, when you reach the stretch position, quickly reverse the movement with a quick twitch of the biceps and begin another rep. Keep your palms facing forward at all times, as this maximizes biceps stretch at the bottom of the movement.

*One-arm nonsupport concentration curls.* Take a dumbbell in one hand and bend at the waist with your arm hanging straight down. Curl the dumbbell up to your shoulder, keeping your torso and upper arm motionless. Flex for two seconds, lower and repeat. Work each arm separately. Try twisting your little finger upward at the top of the movement for a more intense contraction.

*Lying triceps extensions.* Lie on a bench and press a loaded barbell up over your chest with a close grip, leaving about eight inches between your thumbs. Bending your elbows back, lower the bar and touch it to your forehead or to the bench behind your head, whichever is more comfortable. Drive it back over your chest in an arc and repeat without pausing. Some upper-arm movement, which allows the lats to become synergists, is acceptable, as it is a midrange movement.

*Overhead extensions.* These are best done with an EZ-curl bar. Grab the bar, positioning your hands with your thumbs about six inches apart. Press the bar overhead and then lower it back behind your head while keeping your upper arms as stationary as possible. When you reach the stretch position, reverse the movement with a quick triceps twitch and press the bar back overhead. Repeat.

*Kickbacks.* Take a dumbbell in each hand and bend at the waist until your torso is parallel to the floor. With your upper arms next to your sides and your elbows bent at 90 degree angles, extend your forearms back and contract your triceps for two seconds. Your arms should be slightly higher than parallel to the floor in the top position. Lower the dumbbells, keeping your upper arms stationary, and repeat. Tip: Try one set with your palms facing your thighs and one set with your palms facing up. Alternate exercise: one-arm triceps pushdowns.

*Incline wrist curls.* With one end of a bench elevated about four inches, take a close, underhand grip on a loaded barbell and rest your forearms on the high end of the bench with your hands hanging off the end and the angle at your elbows greater than 90 degrees. Curl the bar up until your hands are almost perpendicular to the floor. Lower, and when you reach the stretch position, quickly reverse the movement and repeat.

*Decline wrist curls.* With one end of a bench elevated about four inches, take a close, underhand grip on a loaded barbell and rest your forearms on the low end of the bench with your hands hanging off the end. The angle at your elbows should be less than 90 degrees for best contraction results. Curl the bar up as high as possible and flex your inner forearm muscles for two seconds. Lower and repeat.

*Reverse curls.* Take an overhand, shoulder-width grip on a loaded barbell bar. Stand erect and curl the bar to your shoulders. Lower and repeat. Tip: You can also use an EZ-curl bar on these for a slightly different effect.

*Incline reverse wrist curls.* With one end of your bench elevated about four inches, take a close, overhand grip on a loaded barbell and rest your forearms on the high end of the bench, with your hands hanging off the end and the angle at your elbows greater than 90 degrees. Curl the bar up until your hands are almost perpendicular to the floor. Lower all the way down, then quickly reverse the movement and begin the next rep.

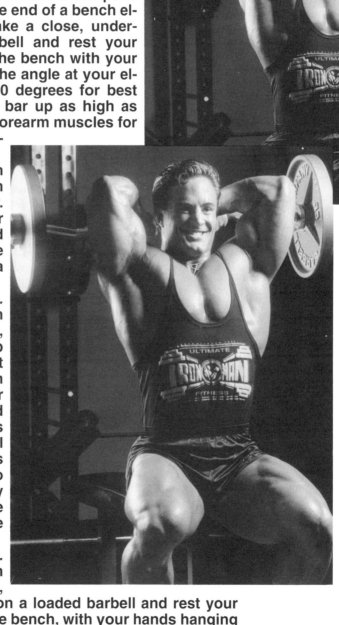

*Decline reverse wrist curls.* With one end of your bench elevated about four inches, take a close, overhand grip on a loaded barbell and rest your forearms on the low end of the bench, with your hands hanging off the end. The angle at your elbows should be less than 90 degrees for best contraction results. Curl the bar up as high as possible and flex your forearm extensors on the tops of your lower arms for two seconds. Lower and repeat.

## Critical Arms Q & A

*Q: I like doing dips and bench dips for my triceps. Neither of these exercises provides resistance in the contracted position even though my arms are down and back at the bottom of both, which fits the contracted-position description. So how do you classify the two exercises?*

*A:* Although there's no resistance in the contracted position, or at least very little, you should still consider both of these exercises contracted-position triceps movements because of the arms-down-and-back finish position you mentioned. As discussed in Chapter 3, the dumbbell flye unofficially qualifies as a contracted-position exercise for the chest for the same reason, so you can substitute dumbbell flyes if you don't have access to a cable crossover apparatus, which provides resistance in the contracted position. If you do use either of the dip exercises as your contracted-position triceps movement, flex hard for a count of two at the top to get a peak-contraction effect, just as you would during dumbbell flyes for the chest. Keep in mind that this isn't as effective as using a contracted-position exercise that has resistance in the finish position, but it's good to use these movements for the sake of variety.

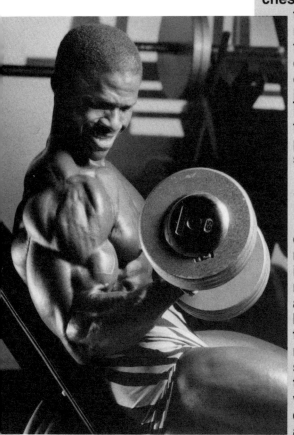

*Q: I really like performing regular pushdowns with a straight bar. Is this a contracted-position exercise for the triceps?*

*A:* Yes, but it's somewhat inferior to one-arm pushdowns and kickbacks because your upper arms can't move behind the plane of your torso to put your triceps in their completely contracted position. You can aproximate this position pretty closely if you use a double-rope attachment, however. If you insist on using a straight bar, go ahead and consider that you're performing a contracted-position movement for your triceps, but incorporate kickbacks and one-arm pushdowns every so often so that you do work your triceps in the completely contracted position. As a side note, if you do pushdowns while bending your torso toward the floor, you turn the exercise into more of a close-grip pressing movement and it falls into the midrange category.

*Q: Although 45-degree-incline dumbbell curls do stretch the biceps, wouldn't a lower incline stretch the muscle farther and thus make it a more effective stretch-position movement?*

*A:* Absolutely. Unfortunately, most trainees don't have the flexibility in their biceps and front delts to go lower than 45 degrees—at first. As your biceps and front delts become accustomed to the 45 degree incline, feel free to go a few notches lower. Don't, however, get too close to a completely horizontal, or flat, position, as you'll place too much strain on your front-delt heads and rotator cuff muscles.

*Q: I like to finish my biceps routine with a double-biceps flex exercise on the cable crossover machine—in the finish position I look as if I'm doing a double-biceps pose. Is this a good contracted-position movement?*

**A:** Yes, you can use it in place of concentration curls as your biceps' contracted-position movement. Because you maintain an outward rotation of your shoulders, though, crossover curls aren't quite as effective as concentration curls for targeting the contracted position. Remember that the biceps' fully contracted position is with your arm overhead and your forearm down and back, as in an overhead triceps extension with your knuckles facing up. In this position your shoulder is rotated in, not out, the way it is when you do the crossover curls. Use the crossover curls for variety's sake, but go back to concentration curls every so often for best results.

*Q: Preacher curls are listed as a midrange exercise for biceps, but there isn't any synergy, or help from other muscle groups, during this movement, so is it really a midrange exercise?*

**A:** While there isn't much synergy during preacher curls, the deltoids are in a partially contracted state, which does help the biceps move the weight. In a strict sense, you're right. The preacher curl lacks true synergy, so only use it once in a while as a midrange movement for your biceps. Stick with regular curls using either dumbbells or a barbell most of the time.

*Q: I use a preacher curl machine that gives me resistance at the top of the movement. Barbell preachers are a midrange-position movement, but they don't have this peak-contraction element. Are machine preachers a midrange- or a contracted-position exercise or both?*

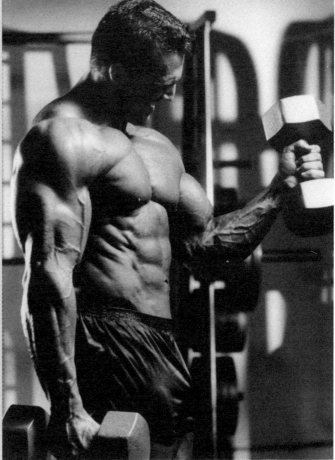

**A:** Although you do get some peak-contraction effect from machine preacher curls, your upper arms aren't far enough forward and away from your body or high enough to achieve the type of contraction you get from concentration curls, where your arm is hanging away from your torso and closer to the biceps' true fully contracted position. If you want to do machine preacher curls, that's fine, but consider them a midrange exercise in spite of the resistance at the top of the movement.

*Q: I like alternating arms on my dumbbell curls. Is this okay?*

**A:** It's fine on all but incline dumbbell curls, which are a stretch-position movement, so you want to take advantage of the prestretch phenomenon in order to engage as many muscle fibers as possible. Incorporating the prestretch twitch at the bottom of each rep is impossible when you're doing alternate incline curls, but on regular dumbbell curls there's no problem.

# CRITICAL ABDOMINALS

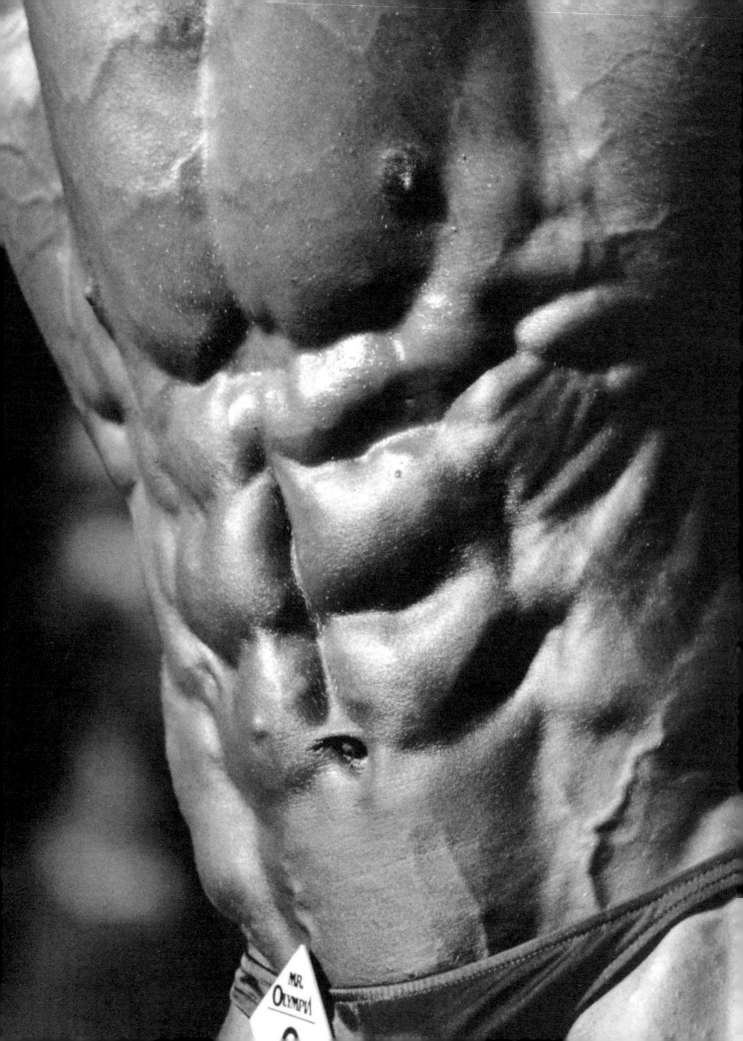

# A New Approach to Rippling Ruggedness

The abdominal area is the focal point of the entire physique as well as a good indicator of whether you're in or out of shape. That's why everyone from models to businesspeople wants a rippling, rugged set of washboard abs. Bodybuilders are especially conscious of chiseling their midsections because it's the first thing contest judges notice in a physique lineup. If the abs aren't developed and delineated to the nth degree, you can bet the athlete will be scored down.

Unfortunately, this emphasis has caused a midsection obsession that may be the very reason why ab training is often such an overdone—and poorly done—effort. Check out any gym and you'll see inexperienced trainees as well as advanced bodybuilders doing hundreds of reps on every midsection exercise known to man with absolutely no method to their madness.

Instead of saddling yourself with a regimen that has you repping till the cows come home, consider the following four facts and then use logic and the Positions-of-Flexion approach to help you overcome your abdominal obstacles:

1) *Muscle makeup.* The abdominal muscles are just that—muscles. Each is made up of the same types of fibers as your biceps, quads and back, not some superfiber that requires extremely high reps—although, because the range of motion is so short on most real ab movements, you may want to do higher reps on certain exercises to get a burn. The abdominal muscle that bodybuilders should be concerned with, the rectus abdominis, is not a bunch of knotted muscle masses, as it appears to be, but rather a sheet-type muscle that runs from the bottom of your rib cage and attaches to your pelvis. The ripples are actually caused by tendons running horizontally and vertically.

2) *Hip flexor function.* The hip flexors come into play on many so-called ab exercises, such as the situp, which makes them inferior to ab isolators like the crunch. The key word here is "isolators." As you'll soon see, the hip flexors are important contributors, or synergists, when you exercise the midrange position of the rectus abdominis.

3) *Upper and lower separation.* The upper rectus abdominis can work independently of the lower part of the muscle, as it does when you perform crunches, but when you work the lower portion, your upper rectus always comes into play, as in reverse crunches or hanging kneeups. Therefore, you should always work the lower area first, which actually brings both upper and lower sections into play. If you isolate the upper part first, when you work your lower abs your upper abs will be fatigued and hamper your lower-ab performance—in much the same way that working forearms before biceps can limit your biceps efforts. For example, if you do crunches first and then hanging kneeups, your upper rectus will be so fatigued from the crunches that it'll cause you to fail on the kneeups long before you fatigue your lower abs.

4) *Efficiency of effort.* You must work your upper and lower abs from the three positions of flexion to get rapid, complete development and delineation.

Because the rectus abdominis can function as two separate muscle groups—as explained in item 3 above—we break down the muscle as follows to

**Critical Mass** 87

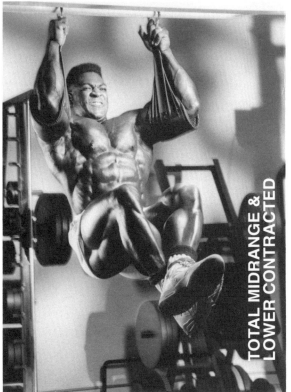

**TOTAL MIDRANGE & LOWER CONTRACTED**

The hanging kneeup is a total-ab midrange movement that brings the hip flexors into play. It's also a lower-ab contracted-position exercise because it provides peak contraction of the lower abs at the top of the movement.

determine its positions of flexion:

### Rectus abdominis (as a whole)

*Midrange:* The midrange movement for the rectus abdominis should involve the hip flexors to a degree. Remember, you're not trying to isolate the target muscle, as a midrange exercise is usually a compound movement that allows surrounding muscles to help the target muscle contract. In this case the hip flexors are the synergists. You work the rectus abdominis through its midrange position with reverse crunches or hanging kneeups.

*Stretch:* The entire rectus abdominis is in the stretch position when your torso is slightly below the plane of your thighs, as in the bottom position of a Roman chair crunch.

### Lower rectus abdominis

*Contracted:* You achieve this position when your upper thighs are almost flush against your abdomen and your hips are rolled upward, as in the finish position of the reverse crunch or hanging kneeup. Note that the reverse crunch and hanging kneeup work the entire rectus abdominis through its midrange position and the lower rectus in its contracted position.

### Upper rectus abdominis

*Contracted:* You hit this position when your upper torso is curled forward toward your pelvis with your hips and lower back remaining on the same plane, as in the standard crunch.

**TOTAL STRETCH**

You hit the abdominals' stretch position when your torso is slightly below the plane of your thighs, as in the bottom of a Roman chair situp.

The upper abdominals' contracted position occurs at the top of a regular crunch.

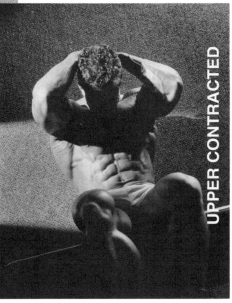

**UPPER CONTRACTED**

With these descriptions rolling around in your mind, you're bound to come up with the perfect POF abdominal workout. To save you brainstorming time—after all, this book is about efficiency—here's the ultimate POF ab routine:

## The POF Abdominal Routine

*Total Midrange & Lower Contracted:*
Reverse crunches, bench kneeups
or hanging kneeups                2 x 10-20
(*Pause at the top for maximum lower-ab contraction, but include little or no pause at the bottom.*)

*Total Stretch:*
Roman chair crunches              2 x 10-20
(*At the bottom, or point of stretch, use a quick twitch for a stronger ab contraction. Also, only go slightly below parallel, as it can be dangerous to stretch the abdominal wall if you're prone to hernias.*)

*Upper Contracted:*
Crunches or cable crunches        1-2 x 10-20
(*Hold at the top of every rep for maximum upper-ab contraction.*)

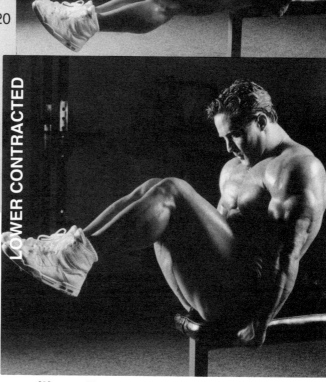

**TOTAL MIDRANGE** — Bench kneeups give you total-ab midrange work and lower-ab contracted work at the top of the movement.

**LOWER CONTRACTED**

Even though you consider the upper and lower rectuses separately, you can still work all three positions of both with only three movements: entire abs' midrange, reverse crunches; entire abs' stretch, Roman chair crunches; upper abs' contracted, crunches. All that's left is the lower abs' contracted position, and you hit that with the first exercise, reverse crunches, along with the entire abs' midrange position. Because of the efficiency, organization and preciseness of the POF approach, this is one of the best regimens for getting a sharply defined midsection. Give it your all and, as long as you keep your bodyfat low, your abs will be the epitome of rippling ruggedness.

Most forms of cable crunches and abdominal machines provide work in only one position, the upper abs' contracted position.

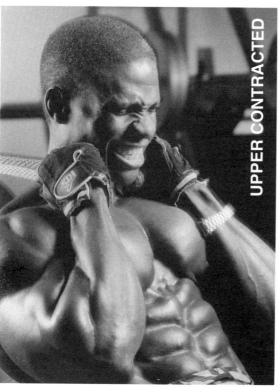

**UPPER CONTRACTED**

## Exercise Descriptions

*Reverse crunches.* Lie on the ground, bend your knees and cross your feet at the ankles. Open your legs until the sides of your thighs are almost touching the floor. With your arms at your sides and hands flat on the ground, curl your knees toward your chest. Your hips will come off the ground a few inches as you "roll up" in the finish position. Exhale and flex your abs for two seconds—remember, this is a lower-ab contracted-position movement as well as a total-ab midrange one. Lower your legs, touch your feet to the floor and repeat. To add resistance, perform the exercise on an incline bench. Alternate exercise: hanging kneeups. Hang from a chinning bar and pull your knees into your chest as you roll your hips toward your torso without any swing. This is a more advanced movement than the reverse crunch, and you'll be able to perform it only if your abs are strong.

*Roman chair crunches.* This is different from the usual Roman chair situp performed in most gyms, which is more of a hip flexor movement. Roman chair crunches take the hip flexors out of the action, although they do receive a stretch along with the abs. Hook your feet under the pads, with your knees bent at approximately 90 degree angles. Lower your torso back until your upper body is just below parallel to the floor and your rectus abdominis is stretched. As soon as you reach this stretch position, reverse your movement and curl your torso up by contracting your abs. The tension should remain on them throughout the rep. Lower and repeat. Be very careful not to go too low on this movement. Some people have weak abdominal walls and are predisposed to tears in this area. If there's a history of hernias in your family, you may want to avoid Roman chair crunches. Alternate exercise: Cable crunches, however this movement doesn't stretch the rectus abdominis as much unless you have some kind of lower-back support.

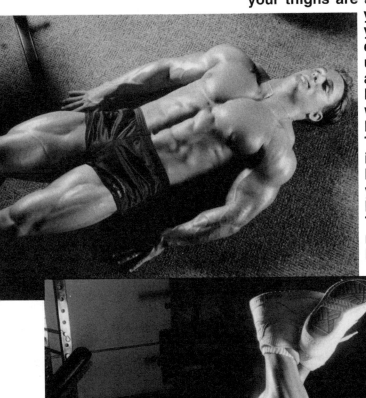

The versitile reverse crunch, a total-ab midrange movement as well as a lower-ab contracted-position exercise.

*Crunches.* Recline on your back on the floor with your lower legs supported on an exercise bench and bent at 90 degree angles to your thighs. Roll up until your upper back is off the floor, blow the air out of your lungs and contract your abs hard for two seconds. Uncurl your body, inhale and repeat. Keep your lower back against the ground at all times.

## Critical Abdominals Q & A

*Q: When I do Roman chair crunches, the abdominal-stretch-position movement, my upper abs feel as if they're getting the same peak contraction they get during regular crunches. Doesn't this mean that Roman chair crunches actually function as both a stretch- and contracted-position exercise?*

*A:* It's difficult for most people to reach the abs' peak-contracted position without the lower-back support you get when you do regular crunches on the floor. Although it may feel as if you're getting a peak contraction at the top of the Roman chair crunches, you're probably not quite reaching it. Even if you are, it's still a good idea to finish off your abs with one set of regular crunches.

*Q: I'm very weak in the abs' stretch position, so I can only manage about three Roman chair crunches. What should I do?*

*A:* Don't give up. When you hit failure, have a partner help you with forced reps until you complete at least eight. Then try to get one more rep on your own at every workout. You'll eventually be able to do eight reps without any help. Also, once you can do 12 reps on your own, go ahead and add weight by placing a barbell plate on your chest. Remember, the abs are just like any other muscle group, and if you want to develop them completely, you have to use progressive resistance.

You can also try a cable crunch movement that will work the stretch and contracted positions. Sit on a preacher bench with the pad supporting your lower back and your back to a cable that's set at head level. Grab the cable handle with both hands—you may want to loop a towel through it for a better grip—and lower back into the stretch position. From there curl forward into the maximum-contracted position. You can also simulate the effect by doing cable crunches with your partner supporting your lower back. Here's an ab routine that incorporates support

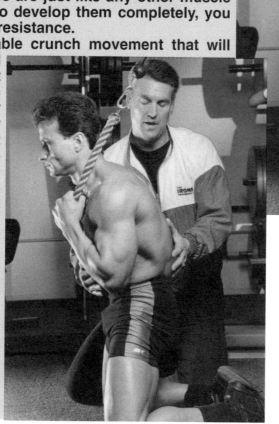

Cable crunches work the upper abs' contracted position (left), and they'll also work the entire rectus abdominis' stretch position—if you have lower-back support, as illustrated above. In these photos Russ Testo is assisted by Fred Koch, creator of the *IRONMAN* Magazine Training System. Note that the cable angles back and is not directly overhead, which ensures resistance in the contracted position.

Critical Mass 91

cable crunches. You can use either variation.

**Total Midrange & Lower Contracted:**
Reverse crunches or hanging kneeups    2 x 10-20

**Total Stretch & Upper Contracted:**
Support cable crunches                  2 x 10-20

This is a very efficient ab program.

*Q: My lower abs are getting strong, and I can do considerably more than 20 reverse crunches, the first POF ab exercise. Should I add some kind of resistance?*

*A:* Yes, you can do them on a situp slant board, placing your head at the high end. The higher you raise the board, the more difficult your reverse crunches will become. You can also substitute hanging kneeups for the reverse crunches, but remember to roll your hips up toward your chest on every rep just as you do on the crunches in order to get the proper effect.

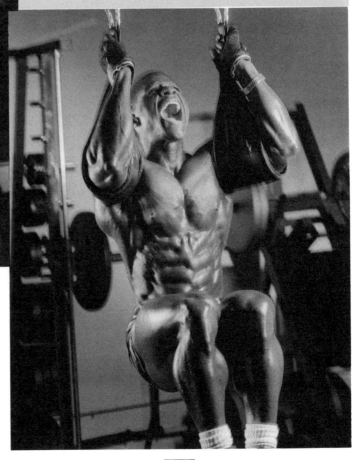

# 8
## POF EVERY-OTHER-DAY SPLIT

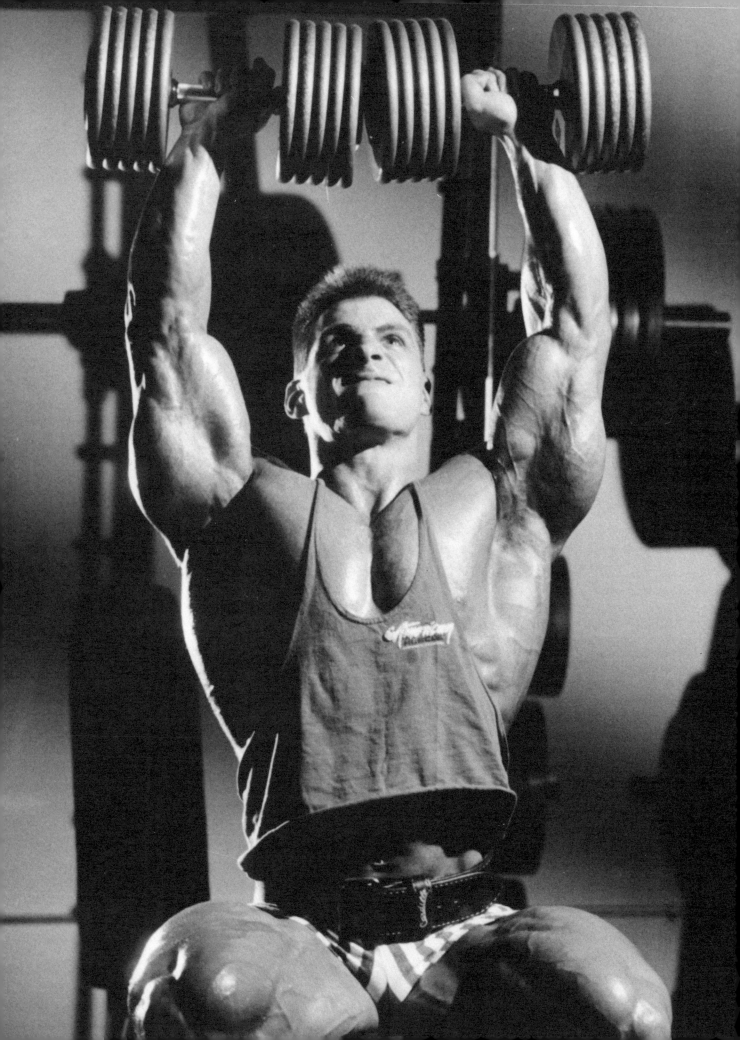

Now that you've seen how the POF method can be applied to all bodyparts, we'll put everything together in a split routine. Before you're ready for this workout, however, you should consider the following points:

1) The standard order for the three positions is midrange first, stretch second and contracted third, and you do them in this order for specific reasons.

• The midrange-position movement works the central bulk of the target muscle with the help of synergist muscles and warms up the target for the more-concentrated work to come in the next two positions.

• In the stretch position you take advantage of the prestretch phenomenon. With a slight twitch, or quick reversal of movement, at the bottom of any stretch-position exercise you can get more power in the full range of motion and thus more fiber involvement. If you work the stretch position first, you increase the possibility of injury because you're stretching a cold muscle. When you work it after the midrange movement, however, the muscle is warm and more capable of stretching and contracting safely.

• The contracted position is where you flex the target muscle with opposing resistance at the point of peak contraction. Movements that hit this position work best if the target muscle is sufficiently warmed up, which is why you usually exercise it last.

2) You can the 1 1/4-reps intensity technique on contracted- and/or stretch-position movements. For example, if concentration curls are your contracted-position biceps movement, flex hard at the top of each rep, lower the dumbbell only 1/4 of the way, then curl it back to the contracted position before lowering to complete extension. This gives you a double-barreled effect in the flexed position. You can do the same thing at the bottom of a stretch-position movement. If, for example, you're performing incline dumbbell curls for biceps, lower the 'bells to complete extension, curl up 1/4 of the way and then lower back to complete extension, where you add a quick twitch to enhance the contraction before curling up again through the full range of motion. Note that you'll have to reduce your poundages when incorporating 1 1/4s on any exercise, but the growth burn you'll get will be incredible.

3) Do at least one light warmup set with 50 percent of your work weight for every midrange movement.

4) Fight the urge to add sets. Two sets is plenty of work for any position, or angle, and one should do it if you're concentrating. A good rule of thumb is to never do more than 25 sets at any one session—and less is preferable. If the routine lists only one set for an exercise but you feel you need two, go ahead and do them, but subtract a set from something else to keep your set total under 25. For example, if you want to do two sets for leg extensions in Workout 1 below, you can either cut your sissy squats to one set or drop a set from another exercise for a strong bodypart. Many people don't like to do this, because they believe that advanced bodybuilders need more sets to keep making gains. This is actually a fallacy, however. The nervous systems of advanced bodybuilders are highly developed through many years of training, so advanced lifters can contract any muscle more intensely. In effect, they can train more efficiently simply because of previously attained neuromuscular development. Advanced bodybuilders don't really need a volume increase over the intermediate workload, only more intensity—they must train harder, not longer.

5) Keep your form strict—two seconds up and two seconds down. The only time you should pick up the speed is at the point of prestretch during a stretch-position movement to improve neurological efficiency—and this should be a quick

> **Advanced bodybuilders don't really need a volume increase, only more intensity—they must train harder, not longer.**

twitch, after which you slow the action once again.

6) With the every-other-day-split routine you train half of your body on one day, rest on the following day, train the other half of your body on the next day and so on. This facilitates recovery, but it also means that you're sometimes training on Saturday or Sunday. Those who don't like to train on the weekends can use the standard four-day split: half on Monday and Thursday and the other half on Tuesday and Friday. This isn't quite as recovery-oriented as the every-other-day split, but it's still quite effective.

7) Always use a phase-training approach; that is, four to six weeks of taking all sets other than warmups to at least positive failure, followed by two weeks of lower-intensity work, stopping all sets two reps short of failure. [See *IRONMAN's Home Gym Handbook* for a complete explanation of phase training.]

8) Although this routine doesn't include forearm work, feel free to add a few sets to the second workout right after you train your biceps if your forearms need extra attention.

9) Review the exercise descriptions in the previous bodypart chapters so you understand the nuances that create the most efficient performance. Sometimes one seemingly insignificant tip can make a world of difference.

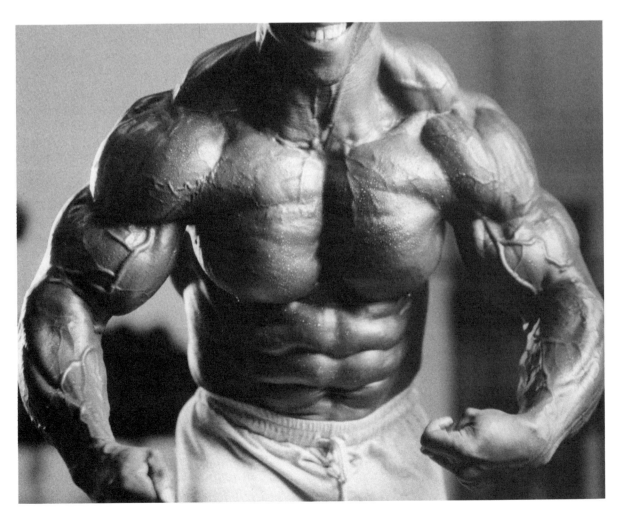

# POF Every-Other-Day Split

**Workout 1**
Quads
   *Midrange:* Squats                                             2 x 8-12
   *Stretch:* Sissy squats                              2 x 8-12
   *Contracted:* Leg extensions                   1 x 8-12
Hamstrings
   *Midrange & Stretch:* Stiff-legged deadlifts    2 x 8-12
   *Contracted:* Lying leg curls                   2 x 8-12
Lower back
   *Contracted:* Hyperextensions                1 x 8-12
Calves
   *Midrange:* Toes-pointed leg curls          1 x 12-20
   *Stretch:* Donkey calf raises                 2 x 12-20
   *Contracted:* Standing calf raises          1 x 12-20
Soleus
   *Contracted:* Seated calf raises            2 x 12-20
Upper chest
   *Midrange:* Incline dumbbell presses     2 x 8-12
   *Stretch & Contracted:* Incline cable flyes  1 x 8-12
Lower chest
   *Midrange:* Barbell bench presses        2 x 8-12
   *Stretch & Contracted:* Decline cable flyes  1 x 8-12
Triceps
   *Midrange:* Lying extensions                2 x 8-12
   *Stretch:* Overhead extensions              1 x 8-12
   *Contracted:* Dumbbell kickbacks          1 x 8-12

**Workout 2**
Midback
   *Midrange:* Behind-the-neck pulldowns   2 x 8-12
   *Stretch & Contracted:* Cable rows       2 x 8-12
Lats
   *Midrange:* Front pulldowns                 2 x 8-12
   *Stretch:* Pullovers                            1 x 8-12
   *Contracted:* Undergrip pulldowns          1 x 8-12
Delts
   *Midrange:* Behind-the-neck presses      2 x 8-12
   *Stretch:* Incline one-arm lateral raises   2 x 8-12
   *Contracted:* Lateral raises                 1 x 8-12
Biceps
   *Midrange:* Barbell curls                       2 x 8-12
   *Stretch:* Incline dumbbell curls             1 x 8-12
   *Contracted:* Concentration curls           1 x 8-12
Abs
   *Midrange & Lower Contracted:* Reverse crunches  1 x 10-20
   *Stretch:* Roman chair crunches           1 x 10-20
   *Upper Contracted:* Crunches                1 x 10-20

# POF HARDGAINER ROUTINE

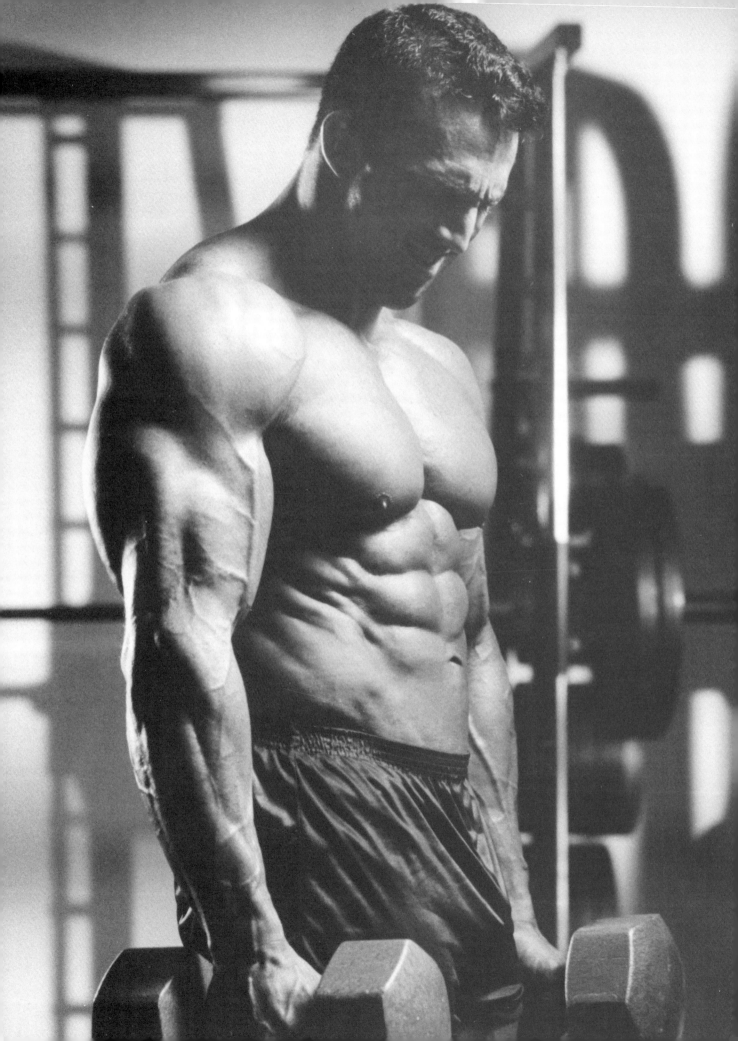

Because bodybuilding is the best way to pack on pounds of muscle, it stands to reason that most of the people who are attracted to lifting weights are skinny ectomorphs with hardgainer tendencies. Of course, not everyone who's skinny is a hardgainer. Take Arnold Schwarzenegger, for example. When he first started lifting weights in his early teens, Arnold had the physique of a bean pole, but after he'd been training for only a few years his musculature revealed the characteristics of a genetic superior.

If you're a skinny individual, don't automatically assume that you fall into the hardgainer category. You could be a natural athlete who simply hasn't blossomed yet. Here's a list of characteristics to look for to determine if you truly are a hardgainer:

1) *Small bones.* Your wrists measure less than 6 3/4 inches.

2) *Unathletic.* Sports and other skilled activities really aren't your thing.

3) *Fast metabolism.* No matter how much you eat, you never put on weight.

4) *Slow muscle growth.* Every pound of muscle is a struggle for you to gain.

5) *High muscle attachments.* When you flex your arm, for example, there's a considerable gap between your lower biceps and your forearm.

If all of the above describes you, the chances are good that you're a hardgainer. Don't let this discourage you, however. You can still make fantastic improvements in muscle size and strength. You just need the right workout, and the following hardgainer POF regimen is one of the best. By adapting the workout from the preceding chapter, which is for athletically inclined mesomorphs, you can gear POF to the hardgainer as well. In fact, POF is one of the best techniques a hardgainer can use, as an adjunct to other strategies such as the 20-rep-squat and power-deadlift routines [see *IRONMAN's Mass-Training Tactics* for more on these techniques], because it completely stimulates the muscles and is recovery oriented.

If you look at the POF Hardgainer Routine listed below, you'll notice that it's quite different from the Every-Other-Day POF Split described in Chapter 8. One important distinction is that the workouts are full-body routines and you only train twice a week. This is to emphasize recovery even more, as most hardgainers take longer to rebound from any type of high-intensity exercise.

You'll also see that midrange exercises are stressed in both the Monday and Friday workouts, while stretch- and contracted-position movements are alternated for most bodyparts at successive sessions. For example, on Monday you work your thighs with squats, a midrange movement, and sissy squats, a stretch-position movement. Then on Friday you do squats again, but this time you follow them with leg extensions, a contracted-position exercise. Because midrange movements are the most efficient for stimulating the bulk of the target muscles, the hardgainer program emphasizes them.

Here are a few other points to keep in mind regarding the Hardgainer POF Routine:

•As mentioned above, you perform midrange exercises at every workout for most bodyparts, after which you either do a stretch- or contracted-position movement. This makes the first session of the week more of a midrange-stretch workout, while the second is more of a midrange-contracted regimen. Each week you work all three positions over two workouts.

•On the day you do leg curls for your hamstrings, you skip toes-pointed leg curls, a midrange movement, for calves. You still work your calves through the midrange to a degree with regular leg curls, but you avoid the more direct calf movement to preserve recovery ability.

•On Monday you work your upper

> **Although POF is more of an advanced technique, hardgainers can still use it with great muscle-building success.**

chest first with incline barbell presses and incline cable flyes, then move on to your lower chest with bench presses. On Friday you reverse the order and train your lower chest first with bench presses and decline cable flyes, then hit your upper chest with incline dumbbell presses. This allows you to work both areas completely and give priority to each once a week without overtraining.

• You flip-flop the order on midback and lats, just as you do on your upper- and lower-chest areas and for the same reasons—priority and recovery. Note also that when you work lats first on Friday, you do front chins, and when you work lats second on Monday you do front pulldowns. This is because when you work lats second your pulling muscles are already fatigued from the midback movement, and pulldowns will allow you to use less than bodyweight if necessary.

• Because of all the indirect stimulation your arms get from pressing and pulling, you don't need to waste recovery ability by training all three positions for biceps and triceps. One exercise apiece will suffice for these muscle groups, and although the routine lists midrange movements, feel free to use a stretch- or contracted-position exercise instead.

• If you add a set somewhere, you may have to subtract a set somewhere else to keep your set total at an acceptable level. Hardgainers should stick to less than 20 per workout.

Remember that although POF is more of an advanced technique, hardgainers can still use it with great muscle-building success. Keep your workouts infrequent—no more than two to three a week—and train hard, and you'll achieve the size and strength you're after.

## Hardgainer POF Routine

**Monday**
Quads
   *Midrange:* Squats — 1 x 8-12
   *Stretch:* Sissy squats — 1 x 8-12
Hamstrings
   *Midrange & Stretch:* Stiff-legged deadlifts — 1 x 8-12
Calves
   *Midrange:* Toes-pointed leg curls — 1 x 12-20
   *Stretch:* Donkey calf raises — 1 x 12-20
Upper chest
   *Midrange:* Incline barbell presses — 1 x 8-12
   *Stretch & Contracted:* Incline cable flyes — 1 x 8-12
Lower chest
   *Midrange:* Bench presses — 1 x 8-12
Midback
   *Midrange:* Behind-the-neck chins — 1 x 8-12
   *Stretch:* V-handle cable rows — 1 x 8-12
Lats
   *Midrange:* Front pulldowns — 1 x 8-12
   *Stretch:* Pullovers — 1 x 8-12
Delts
   *Midrange:* Behind-the-neck presses — 1 x 8-12
   *Stretch:* Incline one-arm lateral raises — 1 x 8-12
Triceps
   *Midrange:* Lying triceps extensions — 1 x 8-12
Biceps
   *Midrange:* Barbell curls — 1 x 8-12
Abs
   *Midrange & Lower Contracted:* Reverse crunches — 1 x 10-20
   *Stretch:* Roman chair crunches — 1 x 10-20

**Friday**
Quads
   *Midrange:* Squats — 1 x 8-12
   *Contracted:* Leg extensions — 1 x 8-12
Hamstrings
   *Midrange & Stretch:* Stiff-legged deadlifts — 1 x 8-12
   *Contracted:* Leg curls — 1 x 8-12
Calves
   *Contracted:* Standing calf raises — 1 x 12-20
Soleus
   *Contracted:* Seated calf raises — 1 x 12-20
Lower chest
   *Midrange:* Bench presses — 1 x 8-12
   *Stretch & Contracted:* Decline cable flyes — 1 x 8-12
Upper chest
   *Midrange:* Incline dumbbell presses — 1 x 8-12
Lats
   *Midrange:* Front chins — 1 x 8-12
   *Contracted:* Stiff-arm pulldowns — 1 x 8-12
Midback
   *Midrange:* Behind-the-neck pulldowns — 1 x 8-12
   *Contracted:* Bent-over lateral raises — 1 x 8-12
Delts
   *Midrange:* Behind-the-neck presses — 1 x 8-12
   *Contracted:* Lateral raises — 1 x 8-12
Triceps
   *Midrange:* Lying triceps extensions — 1 x 8-12
Biceps
   *Midrange:* Barbell curls — 1 x 8-12
Abs
   *Midrange & Lower Contracted:* Reverse crunches — 1 x 10-20
   *Upper Contracted:* Ab machine crunches — 1 x 10-20

# 10 POF POWER PROGRAM

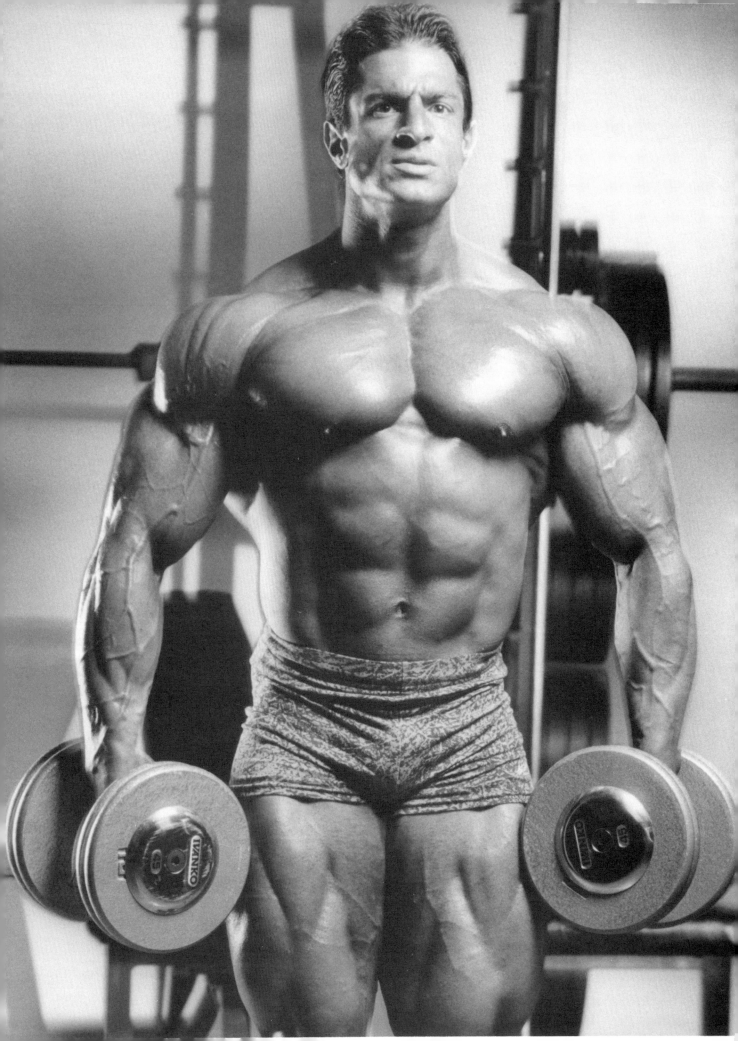

To get big, you have to move heavy iron, and to move heavy iron you have to be strong; so it obviously pays big dividends, literally, to train for strength and power every so often. Unfortunately, some bodybuilders think that training for strength and power means you're forced to neglect proportion and symmetry. Not true. You can train for both simultaneously with the POF Power Program.

This routine is based on the pyramid technique, a poundage-progression method that powerlifters have been using for decades to wring as much strength-building potential out of an exercise as possible. You simply add poundage at each successive set and drop the repetition number accordingly. For example, a powerlifter's bench press workout might look like this:

Set 1   135 x 12
Set 2   185 x 10
Set 3   225 x 8
Set 4   315 x 6
Set 5   350 x 4
Set 6   380 x 2
Set 7   380 x 1-2

As a bodybuilder you want to work the three positions of flexion for complete development while still building plenty of strength. If you use the powerlifter's seven-set pyramid on your midrange movements and then train the other two positions—stretch and contracted—as well, you'll drain too much of your recovery ability, however. Remember that most powerlifters don't care about full, proportionate development, so they don't have to focus on exercises other than the three powerlifts and the assistance movements that help improve those lifts. For bodybuilders, though, it's much better to do a minipyramid on the big midrange exercises and follow each sequence with a stretch- and contracted-position movement for one to two sets in order to avoid doing too much work.

For example, your POF Power Routine for lower chest starts with bench presses for the following set-rep scheme (the poundages are merely hypothetical):

Set 1   135 x 12 (warmup)
Set 2   155 x 10 (warmup)
Set 3   210 x 8
Set 4   235 x 6
Set 5   250 x 3-4

Then you follow this minipyramid progression with one to two all-out sets of decline cable flyes for the stretch and contracted positions of your lower chest. You work every bodypart in a similar manner to build plenty of overall strength without neglecting proportion.

Here are a few tips for making your POF power strategy as productive as possible:

•Do one to two warmup sets with 50 percent of your work weight on each exercise you pyramid. Remember that a warm muscle contracts more efficiently than a cold muscle. (Note that warmup sets are not included in the program outlined below.)

•Whenever you can get 10 reps on the first work set of your power pyramid, up the weight on all three sets at your next workout so that you go back to only getting eight on your first set.

•Go to at least positive failure on all of your sets other than warmups. If you start losing your enthusiasm, however, try a moderate-intensity week; in other words, do four workouts without going to failure. Then on the following week go back to training with all-out intensity.

•Feel free to use intensity techniques like 1 1/4 reps and forced reps, but don't abuse them—never do more than seven to 10 extended sets in any one workout. If you start feeling overtrained, cut back on your use of these techniques immediately. Intensity techniques will probably work best on the stretch- and contracted-position exercises and/or the last set of your pyramid.

[For a detailed description of the best intensity techniques and how to incorporate them for optimal results, see *IRONMAN's Home Gym Handbook*.]

•Take in extra calories, but don't get fat.

If you thought pyramiding was strictly for building strength, think again. Within the powerlifting ranks are some of the most massive athletes in the world, and their size is merely a by-product, or side effect, of their quest for ultimate strength. While it's true that you'll get strong when you pyramid, you'll also build plenty of muscle. If you strive for strength and power, size will follow, and POF will ensure that it's well-porportioned size you're packing on your frame.

> **If you strive for strength and power, size will follow, and POF will ensure that it's well-proportioned size you're packing on your frame.**

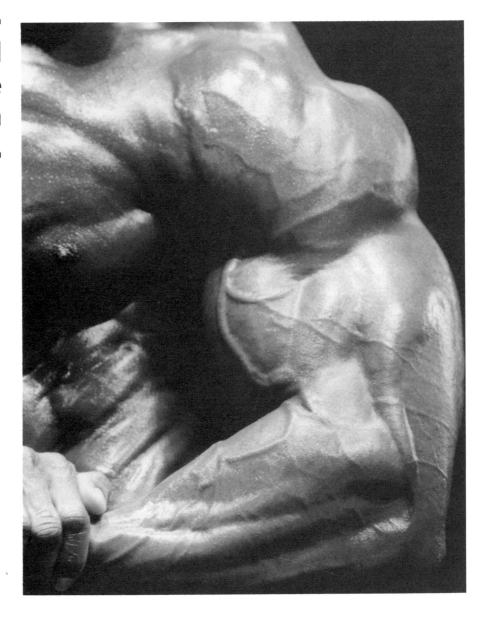

### POF Power Pyramid Program

**Monday & Thursday**
Quads
    *Midrange:* Squats      3 x 8, 6, 3-4
    *Stretch:* Sissy squats      1 x 8-12
    *Contracted:* Leg extensions      1 x 8-12
Hamstrings
    *Midrange & Stretch:* Stiff-legged deadlifts      2 x 8-12
    *Contracted:* Lying leg curls      1 x 8-12
Calves
    *Midrange:* Toes-pointed leg curls      1 x 12-20
    *Stretch:* Donkey calf raises      2 x 12-20
    *Contracted:* Standing calf raises      1 x 12-20
Upper chest
    *Midrange:* Incline Smith machine presses      3 x 8, 6, 3-4
    *Stretch & Contracted:* Incline cable flyes      1 x 8-12
Lower chest
    *Midrange:* Barbell bench presses      3 x 8, 6, 3-4
    *Stretch & Contracted:* Decline cable flyes      1 x 8-12
Triceps
    *Midrange:* Close-grip bench presses      3 x 8, 6, 3-4
    *Stretch:* Overhead extensions      1 x 8-12
    *Contracted:* Dumbbell kickbacks      1 x 8-12

**Tuesday & Friday**
Midback
    *Midrange:* Behind-the-neck pulldowns      3 x 8, 6, 3-4
    *Stretch & Contracted:* One-arm dumbbell rows      1 x 8-12
Lats
    *Midrange:* Front pulldowns      3 x 8, 6, 3-4
    *Stretch:* Pullovers      1 x 8-12
    *Contracted:* Stiff-arm pulldowns      1 x 8-12
Delts
    *Midrange:* Behind-the-neck presses      3 x 8, 6, 3-4
    *Stretch:* Incline one-arm lateral raises      1 x 8-12
    *Contracted:* Lateral raises      1 x 8-12
Biceps
    *Midrange:* Barbell curls      3 x 8, 6, 3-4
    *Stretch:* Incline dumbbell curls      1 x 8-12
    *Contracted:* Concentration curls      1 x 8-12
Abs
    *Midrange & Lower Contracted:* Reverse crunches      1 x 10-20
    *Stretch:* Roman chair crunches      1 x 10-20
    *Upper Contracted:* Crunches      1 x 10-20
Soleus
    *Contracted:* Seated calf raises      3 x 12, 10, 6-8

# 11 POF TARGET OVERLOAD

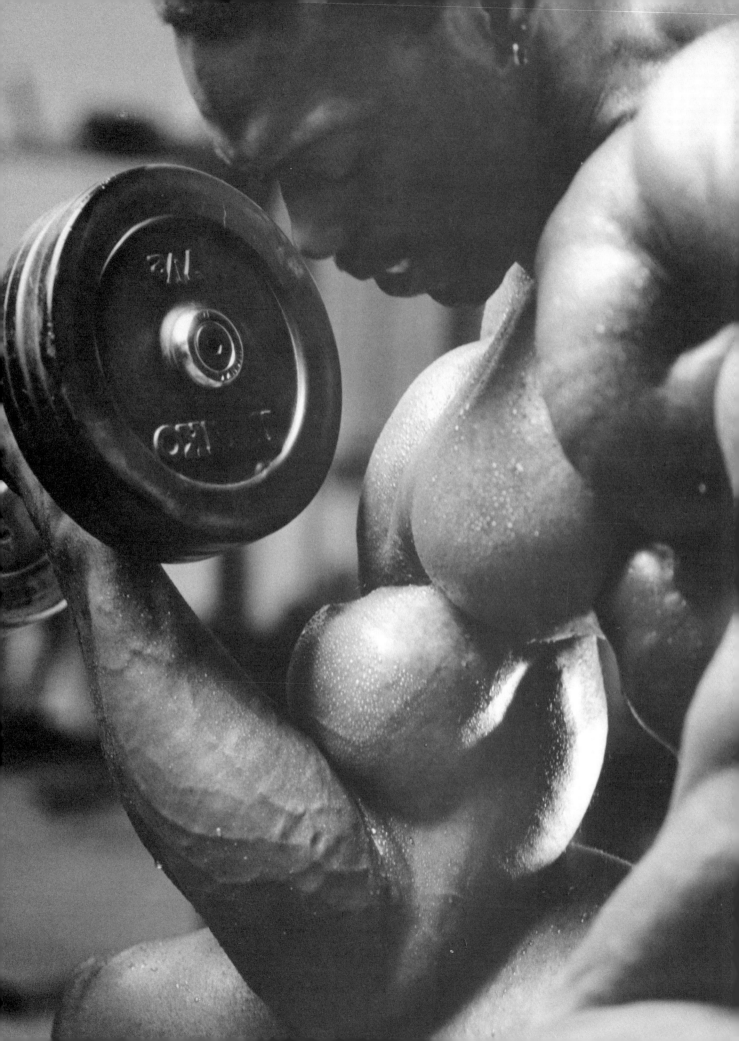

Target-overload training is a method of intentionally overtraining each target muscle group and then giving it an entire week to recover from its overly depleted state. You can best accomplish this by upping the volume for each muscle group and training your entire body over five workouts. This one-to-two-bodyparts-per-day regimen is becoming increasingly popular in the pro bodybuilding ranks because it allows trainees to quench their thirst for more work while still getting enough recovery time. Steve Brisbois, a former World Amateur champion and a successful IFBB pro, claims that this approach helped him get fuller and harder because of the enhanced recuperation.

The reason this strategy is so effective is because not only do you give each muscle group up to a week of recovery time before you bombard it with direct work again, but you also get a mental boost knowing that you only have to train one or two bodyparts when you hit the iron. The concentrated focus gives you the mental and physical energy to really pour on the intensity and overload the target muscles every time. Combine this target-overload tactic with POF, and you have one powerful mass-building strategy.

Here are a few things to consider when using the POF Target Overload routine:

- Each session should contain no more than 25 sets.

- Each workout should take no more than approximately 45 minutes.

- Hit each bodypart with nine to 10 sets.

- Give every set other than warmups your all and take it to at least positive failure, incorporating intensity techniques, such as forced reps, every so often. You're only directly training each bodypart once a week, so you can really let go.

Here's how you split things up:

*Monday:* Delts & calves
*Tuesday:* Lats, midback & hamstrings
*Wednesday:* Chest & upper traps
*Thursday:* Quadriceps & abs
*Friday:* Biceps, triceps & forearms

Remember that your goal is to overload—and, therefore, slightly overtrain—each bodypart. Because an entire seven days passes before a particular muscle group is directly stimulated again, your bodyparts get ample time to recover from this overtrained state, they adapt to the overload, and they grow.

Another thing that makes the routine so effective is the indirect effect. Bodyparts are indirectly stimulated on days when they don't get direct work because they act either as stabilizers—muscles that hold your body in position so you can perform a movement, such as the way the abdominals assist during squats—or synergists—muscles that contribute directly to the movement, such as they way the triceps work during overhead presses.

For example, you work your delts directly on Monday, but they get indirect work from chest training on Wednesday and biceps training on Friday. This indirect stimulation helps facilitate recovery by removing waste products from the deltoids that were created by the direct overload on Monday.

Because of these size-and-strength-building benefits, target-overload training is worth using every so often in your quest for size. It will bring you an overabundance of muscle stimulation and adaption, which translates into more-massive muscles.

### POF Target Overload

**Monday**
Delts
   *Midrange:* Behind-the-neck presses — 3 x 8-10
   *Stretch:* Incline one-arm lateral raises — 3 x 8-10
   *Contracted:* Lateral raises — 3 x 8-10
Calves
   *Midrange:* Toes-pointed leg curls — 2 x 12-20
   *Stretch:* Leg press calf raises — 3 x 12-20
   *Contracted:* Standing calf raises — 3 x 12-20
Soleus
   *Contracted:* Seated calf raises — 3 x 12-20

**Tuesday**
Midback
   *Midrange:* Behind-the-neck chins — 3 x 8-10
   *Stretch & Contracted:* Bent-over rows — 3 x 8-10
Lats
   *Midrange:* Front pulldowns — 3 x 8-10
   *Stretch & Contracted:* Machine pullovers — 3 x 8-10
Hamstrings
   *Midrange & Stretch:* Stiff-legged deadlifts — 3 x 8-10
   *Contracted:* Leg curls — 3 x 8-10
Lower back
   *Contracted:* Hyperextensions — 3 x 8-10

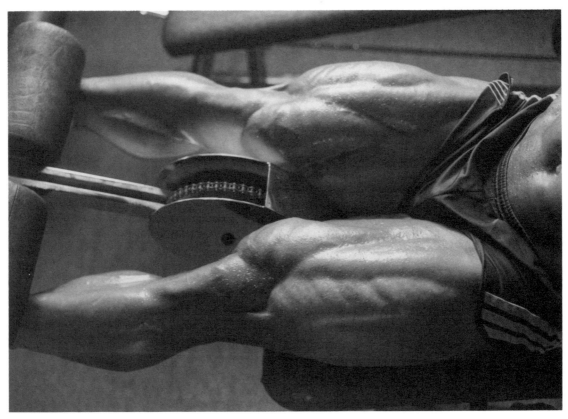

### Wednesday
Upper chest
- *Midrange:* Incline presses — 3 x 8-10
- *Stretch:* Incline dumbbell flyes — 2 x 8-10
- *Contracted:* Low-cable crossovers — 2 x 8-10

Lower chest
- *Midrange:* Bench presses — 3 x 8-10
- *Stretch:* Flat-bench flyes — 2 x 8-10
- *Contracted:* Pec deck flyes — 2 x 8-10

Upper traps
- *Stretch & Contracted:* Forward-lean shrugs — 3 x 8-10

### Thursday
Quads
- *Midrange:* Squats — 3 x 8-10
- *Stretch:* Sissy squats — 3 x 8-10
- *Contracted:* Leg extensions — 3 x 8-10

Abs
- *Midrange & Lower Contracted:* Hanging kneeups — 3 x 10-20
- *Stretch:* Roman chair crunches — 3 x 10-20
- *Upper Contracted:* Crunches or cable crunches — 3 x 10-20

### Friday
Biceps
- *Midrange:* Alternate dumbbell curls — 3 x 8-10
- *Stretch:* Incline dumbbell curls — 2 x 8-10
- *Contracted:* Concentration curls — 2 x 8-10

Triceps
- *Midrange:* Lying extensions — 3 x 8-10
- *Stretch:* One-arm overhead dumbbell extensions — 2 x 8-10
- *Contracted:* Kickbacks — 2 x 8-10

Forearm flexors
- *Stretch:* Incline wrist curls — 1 x 8-12
- *Contracted:* Decline wrist curls — 1 x 8-12

Forearm extensors
- *Midrange:* Hammer curls — 1 x 8-12
- *Stretch:* Incline reverse wrist curls — 1 x 8-12
- *Contracted:* Decline reverse wrist curls — 1 x 8-12

# 12
## POF PRE-EXHAUSTION

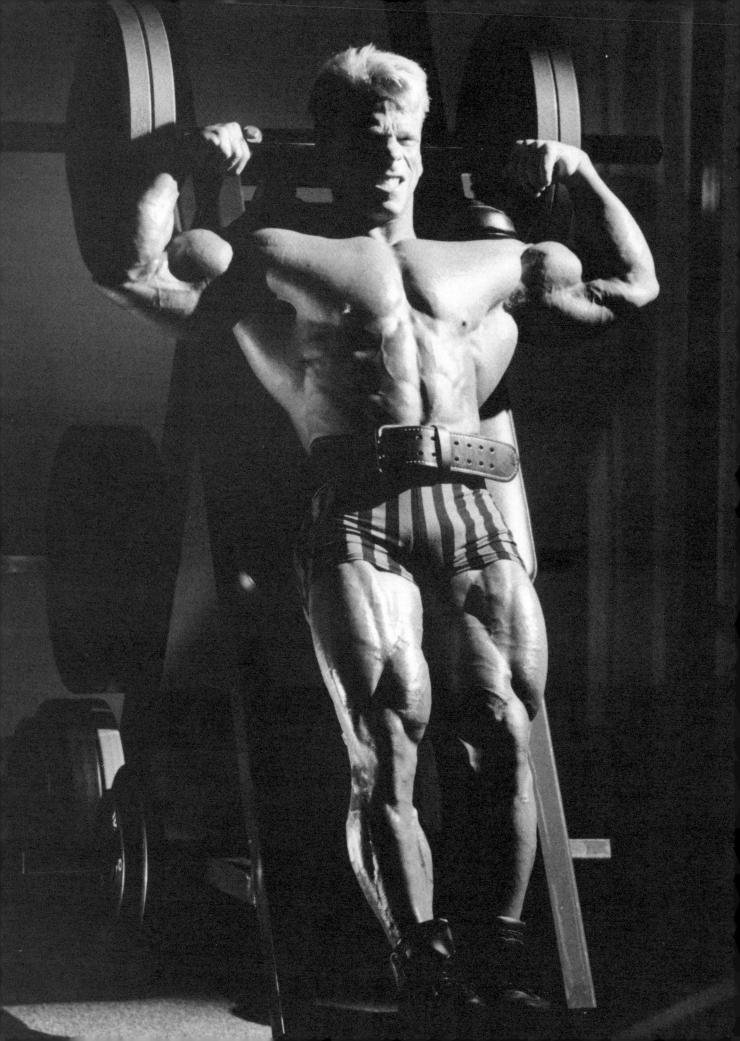

Intensity is the primary prerequisite for muscle growth. The harder you train a muscle, the more likely it is to overcompensate by getting bigger. Unfortunately, hitting a muscle with direct, intense stress can be difficult with conventional training methods due to what are known as weak links.

A weak link is simply a smaller bodypart that limits the work of a larger bodypart during certain exercises. For example, when you bench-press, your smaller triceps fatigue before your larger, stronger pectorals, which means that your pecs don't get nearly as much direct stimulation as they should. Most bodybuilders try to counter this by doing more sets, but, as you know, adding work is definitely the wrong approach if you want to preserve your recovery ability and avoid overtraining.

The best method for overcoming this weak-link problem is pre-exhaustion, a muscle-shocking technique that can give you large size increases—if you use it judiciously. This is such an excellent growth stimulator that Nautilus built it into almost all of its machines at great engineering expense.

You don't need Nautilus machines to take advantage of pre-exhaustion, however. You can use conventional equipment and still reap the mass-building rewards. Pre-exhaustion is not a difficult concept to grasp: You simply eliminate the weak link by immediately following an isolation exercise with a compound exercise for that same bodypart.

To use the example discussed above, when you perform the bench press, your smaller, weaker triceps give out before you exhaust your pectorals. To get around this you prefatigue the target muscles, in this case the pecs, with an isolation exercise, such as cable crossovers, before you do your compound movement, the bench press. This temporarily weakens your target muscle group, in this case the chest, and gives the weak link a strength advantage in order to help push the target to the limit.

Here's an example of how to do a pre-exhaustion set for your deltoids, where the triceps again are the weak link.

Grab a pair of dumbbells and crank out a set of lateral raises. The weight should be heavy enough that you can only get six to eight strict reps. This set will thoroughly fatigue your side-delt heads. Now, immediately after you finish the laterals, take a loaded barbell—lighter than what you usually use on this exercise—and push out a set of behind-the-neck presses. This will force your delts to continue to work with the help of the stronger—for the moment—triceps.

If you were to do the behind-the-neck presses first, as most trainees do, your triceps would give out before your stronger deltoids, in which case your delts wouldn't really be working to failure. Weak links are prevalent in almost all compound, or multi-joint, exercises. Here's a list of the major bodyparts, their corresponding compound movements and the weak links involved:

*Thighs*
  Squats, lower back
*Hamstrings*
  Stiff-legged deadlifts, lower back
*Deltoids*
  Behind-the-neck presses, triceps
*Chest*
  Bench presses, triceps
*Lats*
  Chins or pulldowns, biceps
*Midback*
  Rows, biceps

Although Robert Kennedy, publisher of *MuscleMag International*, is considered to be the creator of pre-exhaustion, it was Mike Mentzer who showed what it could do. With it he won the Mr. Universe and successfully competed at the pro level for many years—and because his training was so intense, he was able to finish his workouts in about one-third the time it took his competitors. They lasted only 45 minutes to an hour, and he trained four days per week. Mentzer used pre-exhaustion throughout his bodybuilding career and made tremendous gains with very brief workouts. The question is, Is it pos-

> **POF Pre-ex really jolts every muscle to its core, and with it you'll realize what real pain zone training is all about.**

sible to improve on pre-exhaustion and make it even better than the version Mentzer used? The answer is yes—by combining it with an efficient multi-angular training method like POF.

With the POF Pre-ex Routine you not only eliminate weak links, but you also work each muscle group through its three positions of flexion. This really jolts every muscle to its core, but because of the to-the-bone shock you shouldn't use POF Pre-ex for more than a few weeks at a time. Beginners and early intermediates should avoid it completely.

The ideal POF Pre-ex cycle has you start out with a contracted-position movement because that type of isolation exercise causes an intense contraction in the target muscle's flexed position without giving it any rest—there's resistance throughout the entire range of motion. When you finish the exercise, you move immediately to a midrange movement to take advantage of the temporarily stronger weak link. After one or two of these supersets you finish off the bodypart with one to two sets of a stretch-position exercise, which incorporates the prestretch phenomenon.

Look at the routine in this chapter, and you'll see that the majority of bodyparts are trained according to this protocol. Of course, there are exceptions, but many of them actually make the pre-exhaustion method more advantageous and efficient. For example, the hamstrings workout consists of leg curls, a contracted-position movement, followed by stiff-legged deadlifts, a combination midrange- and stretch-position exercise. The two-positions-in-one exercises make pre-ex that much more effective because you fatigue more of the muscle in less time.

Once you try POF Pre-ex, you'll immediately see why it's one of the best techniques for upping your muscle mass, and you'll realize what real pain zone training is all about. Be prepared.

Here are a few tips for using pre-exhaustion:

•Don't rest between the contracted-position and midrange-position exercises.

•Always keep the weight under control—no jerking or writhing around to get an extra rep.

•Never do more than two pre-exhaustion cycles for a particular bodypart; one is usually plenty. A good rule is to do two pre-ex cycles for your weaker bodyparts and only one for your stronger bodyparts. Always pay attention to your set total, however, which shouldn't exceed 25.

•Use the routine on an every-other-day-split schedule: Workout 1 on Monday; rest on Tuesday; Workout 2 on Wednesday; rest on Thursday; Workout 1 on Friday; and so on.

•Don't use POF Pre-ex for more than three to four weeks straight. You must respect this method's awesome intensity capabilites, or you'll undoubtedly overtrain and regress.

## POF Pre-ex Routine

**Workout 1**
Quads
   *Contracted:* Leg extensions — 1-2 x 8-12
      *cycled with*
   *Midrange:* Squats — 1-2 x 8-12
   *Stretch:* Sissy squats — 1 x 8-12
Hamstrings
   *Contracted:* Lying leg curls — 1 x 8-12
      *cycled with*
   *Midrange & Stretch:* Stiff-legged deadlifts — 1-2 x 8-12
Lower back
   *Contracted:* Hyperextensions — 1-2 x 8-12
Calves
   *Contracted:* Standing calf raises — 1-2 x 12-20
      *cycled with*
   *Midrange:* Toes-pointed leg curls — 1-2 x 12-20
   *Stretch:* Donkey calf raises — 2 x 12-20
Soleus
   *Contracted:* Seated calf raises — 1 x 12-20
Upper chest
   *Stretch & Contracted:* Incline cable flyes — 1-2 x 8-12
      *cycled with*
   *Midrange:* Incline dumbbell presses — 1-2 x 8-12
Lower chest
   *Stretch & Contracted:* Decline cable flyes — 2 x 8-12
      *cycled with*
   *Midrange:* Barbell bench presses — 2 x 8-12
Triceps*
   *Contracted:* Kickbacks — 1 x 8-12
      *cycled with*
   *Midrange:* Close-grip bench presses — 1 x 8-12
   *Stretch:* Overhead extensions — 1 x 8-12

*The triceps aren't hampered by weak links, but by pre-exhausting them with an isolation exercise you can force them to work harder with a compound movement that elicits the help of a stronger bodypart. In this routine the chest helps the triceps during close-grip bench presses.

**Workout 2**
Midback
   *Contracted:* Bent-arm bent-over lateral raises — 1-2 x 8-12
      *cycled with*
   *Midrange:* Behind-the-neck pulldowns — 1-2 x 8-12
   *Stretch:* V-handle cable rows — 1 x 8-12
Lats
   *Contracted:* Stiff-arm pulldowns — 1-2 x 8-12
      *cycled with*
   *Midrange:* Front pulldowns — 1-2 x 8-12
   *Stretch:* Pullovers — 1 x 8-12
Delts
   *Contracted:* Lateral raises — 1-2 x 8-12
      *cycled with*
   *Midrange:* Behind-the-neck presses — 1-2 x 8-12
   *Stretch:* Incline one-arm lateral raises — 1-2 x 8-12
Biceps*
   *Contracted:* Spider curls — 1 x 8-12
      *cycled with*
   *Midrange:* Undergrip pulldowns — 1 x 8-12
   *Stretch:* Incline dumbbell curls — 1 x 8-12
Abs
   *Upper Contracted:* Crunches — 1 x 10-20
      *cycled with*
   *Midrange & Lower Contracted:* Reverse crunches — 1 x 10-20
   *Stretch:* Roman chair crunches — 1 x 10-20

*The biceps aren't hampered by weak links, but by pre-exhausting them with an isolation exercise you can force them to work harder with a compound movement that elicits the help of a stronger bodypart. In this routine the back pushes the biceps during undergrip pulldowns.

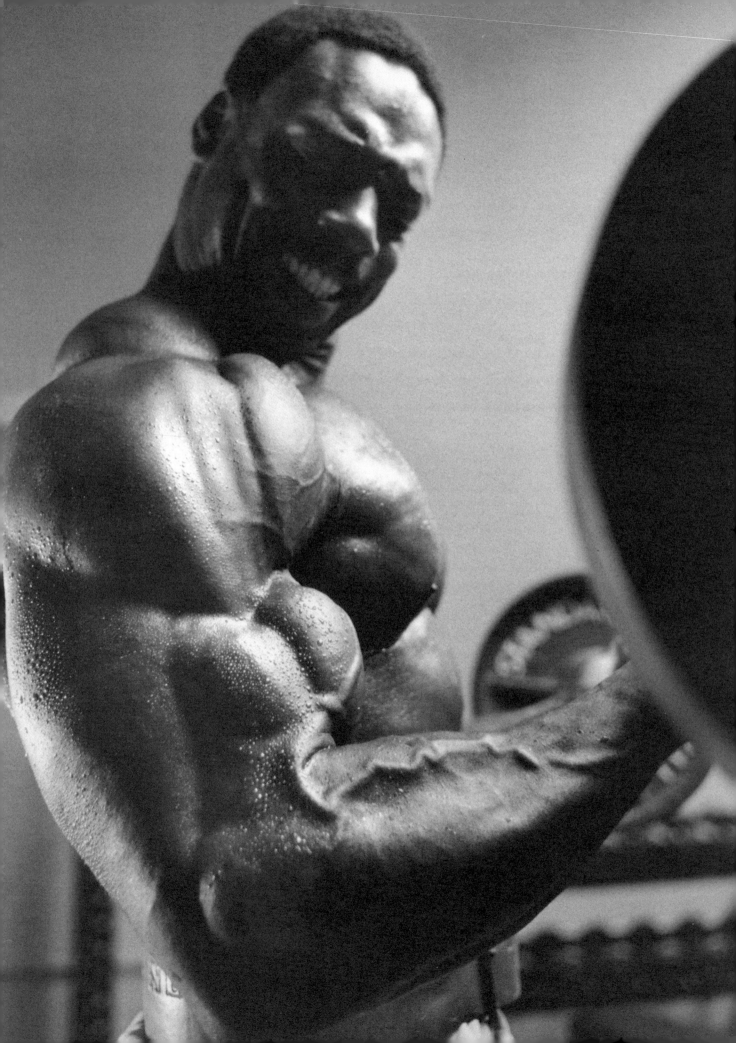

# AFTERWORD

Although POF is one of the best bodybuilding methods available, it won't build an ounce of muscle without sheer, unadulterated effort. You've got to pour all the intensity you can muster into the routines in this book if you want them to push your physique to new levels of massiveness.

You can't be afraid of all-out effort. You build size by overloading your muscles. Load them with intensity over and above what you did previously and allow enough recovery time, and they'll grow larger and stronger; keep this overload coming at a steady rate, and you'll eventually achieve your dream of incredible size and strength.

With consistent, intense, intelligent training you'll make the most rapid bodybuilding gains possible and eventually attain the desire of every lifter in every gym the world over—critical mass. POF can help you achieve this dream.

Train efficiently and effectively, and you'll reach your ultimate bodybuilding goals. Good luck.

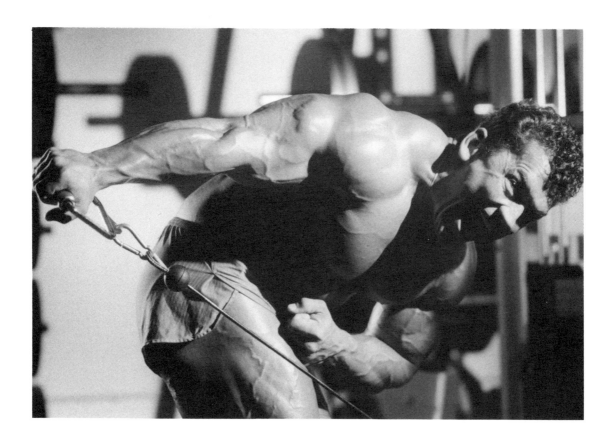

# OTHER POWER-PACKED *IRONMAN* PRODUCTS

### *IRONMAN's* HOME GYM HANDBOOK
*A Complete Guide to Training at Home*

This book shows you how to get huge in your own home. It has details on how to set up your own home gym as well as information on intensity, recovery and bodypart specialization. It also includes many supereffective muscle-building routines and tips, including the first POF routine.

by Steve Holman

**$14.95**

### *COMPOUND AFTERSHOCK*
*POF Update 1*

Move up the POF ladder of intensity with Compound Aftershock training and the Compound Aftershock routine. This book also includes the Supercompensation workout, Isolation Aftershock training and the Double-Impact technique.

by Steve Holman

**$14.95**

### *IRONMAN's* MASS-TRAINING TACTICS
*Size-Building Strategies for Home- or Commercial-Gym Bodybuilders*

More than 20 complete mass-boosting routines, including Pre-Exhaustion, Target Overload, the Supersize Superset Strategy, Anabolic Acceleration and the Power Pyramid. This is *real* bodybuilding at its best!

by Steve Holman

**$14.95**

### *IRONMAN BULLETIN #1: 10-WEEK SIZE SURGE*
*A Crash Course for Packing On Muscle Weight*

This bulletin includes two high-intensity-training phases built into a 10-week cycle, the Size Surge Diet, a balanced meal-by-meal eating schedule with the perfect protein, carb and fat percentages that deliver accelerated anabolic uptake and the 7 Sacred Rules for Packing On Muscle Weight You Should Never Break. One man gained 20 pounds of muscle on this exact program in only 10 weeks and added 1 1/2 inches to his arms!

by Steve Holman

**$9.95**

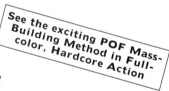

### *IRONMAN's* "CRITICAL ARMS" VIDEO
*Live-action POF Biceps, Triceps and Forearm Training*

**$24.95**

### *IRONMAN's* "CRITICAL CHEST & DELTS" VIDEO
*Live-action POF Pec and Shoulder Training*

**$24.95**

### *IRONMAN's* "CRITICAL LEGS & BACK" VIDEO
*Live-action POF Quad, Hamstring, Calf and Back Training*

**$24.95**

### *SPECIAL OFFER*
Get all three POF videos for only *$49.95 (you save $25)*

To order by credit card call **1-800-447-0008, ext. 1**
or send check or money order for the amount plus $3.50 shipping and handling for each book or $4.50 for each video to

*IRONMAN* Products, 1701 Ives Ave., Oxnard, CA 93033

# Move Up the Ladder of Intensity
## And Take Your Mass to the Next Level

It's time to jolt your muscles to startling new levels of size with **Compound Aftershock**. Here is the latest muscle-building research centered around the exciting Positions-of-Flexion mass-boosting method that has been getting rave reviews from bodybuilders worldwide. **POF produces radical results and an unreal skin-stretching pump at every workout** because of its powerful maximum-fiber recruitment capabilities. In this research update you'll learn how to take your workouts up the ladder of intensity and how certain exercise techniques and combinations can pack dramatic new muscle mass on your frame by activating an **even higher level of fiber recruitment**—and **with only three to four sets per bodypart!** Finally you can ignite your training intensity to blast-furnace levels without burning out. If you've read *Critical Mass* and have tried POF for six months, you're ready for more **shocking gains in size and strength.** *Compound Aftershock* will help you push your mass to the next level.

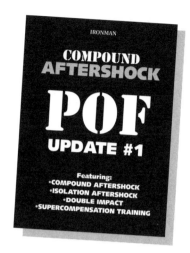

With this exciting new manual you'll discover:

- **The Compound Aftershock and Isolation Aftershock techniques and routines.** Blast even more fibers out of reserve with these powerful ultra-intensity methods.

- **Supercompensation.** Train each bodypart only once a week for super size gains.

- **Double-Impact training.** How you can infuse certain exercises with two to three times more mass acceleration.

- **The Power of POF.** More on how this powerful method can up your gains to levels you thought were impossible.

- **The POF Exercise Grid.** An in-the-gym exercise reference for each bodypart that lists the positions of flexion movements.

### Just $14.95

plus $3.50 postage & handling ($5 outside North America) (California residents add 8.25% sales tax)

*Credit card orders call*

### 1-800-447-0008, ext.1
### (24-hour order line)

---

❏**YES!** I want to take my mass to new levels with *Compound Aftershock—POF Update #1.* Rush it to me immediately.

Rush my copy to: ........................................................
........................................................
........................................................

Enclose check or money order for $14.95 plus $3.50 S&H payable to:

Homebody Productions
P.O. Box 2800
Ventura, CA 93002

**Credit card orders call TOLL FREE 1-800-447-0008, ext.1**

CA residents add 8.25% sales tax. Foreign orders (except Canada) $5 shipping. Payment in U.S. dollars drawn on U.S. banks only.